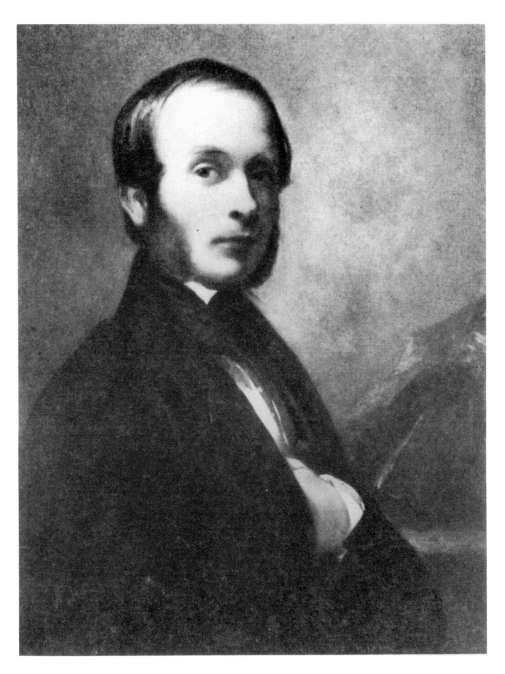

Dr John Snow (1813–1858), as a young man

ON NARCOTISM BY THE INHALATION OF VAPOURS

by

JOHN SNOW

A facsimile edition
with an introductory essay

by

RICHARD H ELLIS

MB, BS, D Obst, RCOG, FFARCS, FC Anaes

Consultant Anaesthetist, The Royal Hospital of
Saint Bartholomew, London, UK

Honorary Consultant Anaesthetist, Queen Charlotte's
Hospital, London, UK

Royal Society of Medicine Services Limited

Royal Society of Medicine Services Limited
1 Wimpole Street   London W1M 8AE
7 East 60th Street   New York NY 10022

British Library Cataloguing in Publication Data
Snow, John, *1813–1858*
On narcotism by the inhalation of vapours.
 I. Title
 615.72

 ISBN 1-85315-158-0

Phototypeset by Dobbie Typesetting Limited, Tavistock, Devon
Printed in Great Britain by Whitstable Litho, Whitstable, Kent.

To the memory of

Dr Monica Cronin

1933–1990

Acknowledgements

The publication of this facsimile edition would not have been possible without the practical help which Miss Joan Ferguson, the Librarian of The Royal College of Physicians of Edinburgh, gave so willingly. I am most grateful to her, and to the College's Library Committee, for allowing me to use their copies of John Snow's pamphlets in the preparation of this volume.

I am indebted to Dr Geoffrey Snow for permitting me to use, as a frontispiece, the portrait of John Snow as a young man. This is taken from the oil painting which is now in his possession. The photograph is reproduced by kind permission of the Editor of the *Journal of The Royal Society of Medicine*.

It is a pleasure to acknowledge the assistance which I have received from Howard Croft, Brian Weight, Helen McKay and Delia Siedle of the Publications Department at The Royal Society of Medicine. Howard Croft willingly adopted the project as soon as he became aware of its significance; this is not the first time that he has enhanced the literature of the history of Anaesthesia, and I hope it will not be the last.

Contents

Introduction

In chronological order, Snow's most renowned publications are *On the Inhalation of the Vapour of Ether in Surgical Operations* (published in 1847),[1] the second edition of *On the Mode of Communication of Cholera* (published in 1855),[2] and *On Chloroform and other Anaesthetics: their Action and Administration* (published in 1858 shortly after his death).[3] Original or first editions of each of these works are extremely rare, and several facsimile versions have been produced. For example, Snow's 1847 treatise on ether has been reproduced in facsimile form no less than four times[4-7] and his works on chloroform and on the spread of cholera at least once each.[8,9] The reprinting of these original texts has focused attention away from his many other writings on medicine and related topics. There are many of these, and there is, as yet, no comprehensive bibliography of Snow's contributions to the medical literature.

In May 1848, within eighteen months of anaesthesia's introduction to Britain, John Snow began to write a sequence of eighteen remarkable articles entitled *On Narcotism by the Inhalation of Vapours*. They were initially published in serial form in the *London Medical Gazette* over the next three and a half years.[10-27] The articles were also assembled for publication in pamphlet form. The first seven were published together,[28] as were the next nine,[29] and then the last two.[30] The resulting three pamphlets, reproduced in this edition, were not merely collections of reprints for there are separate title pages and lists of contents, and their pagination differs from that found in the journal itself. However, it would appear that the blocks were kept by the printers and used to prepare both versions, although a few typographical corrections and other minor changes were made to the journal's text prior to the printing of the pamphlets. This indicates that the decision to reprint the series in a collected form was taken (presumably by Snow himself) right at the outset. Unfortunately, none of the pamphlets has a preface to indicate the purpose which Snow had in mind for the reprinted work. The pamphlets were produced in London by the printers of the *London Medical Gazette,* and it is likely that Snow published them privately for no formal publishing house was involved.

Few of the individual pamphlets have survived, and a complete, three volume set of the reprinted version of *On Narcotism by the Inhalation of Vapours* seems to be extremely rare indeed. The pamphlets have been incompletely catalogued both in the United States and in Britain. The *British Museum General Catalogue of Printed Books*[31] does not list them at all, and the *Index Catalogue of the Library of the Surgeon-General's Office* (in the United States)[32] lists the first two pamphlets but makes no mention of the third. All three of the pamphlets are listed in the American *National Union Catalog*.[33] A search conducted by the British Library indicated that no complete set would be found in any of the relevant major research libraries in the English-speaking world. Eventually, however, one was located in the Library of the Royal College of Physicians of Edinburgh. It would seem that no others exist, although the publication of this facsimile edition may serve as a stimulus which brings more to light.

The three separate pamphlets appeared at unpredictable intervals, in 1848,[28] 1851[29] and 1852,[30] and this reflects the irregular pattern of the times at which the original articles were published in the journal. The first seven instalments (which, on average, had been published at the rate of one part a month) were produced as a pamphlet soon after the seventh article had appeared in the *London Medical Gazette* on the 17 November 1848.[16] This had ended with a detailed and illustrated description of the latest version of Snow's chloroform inhaler (p 34). Presumably the issuing of the first pamphlet, at this stage, would have helped Snow to publicise this inhaler as widely and as soon as possible. Parts eight to sixteen were published as the second pamphlet in 1851. They had appeared in the journal between mid-December 1848[17] and April 1851[25] at an average rate of one every three and a half months—although there were two long gaps in this sequence, the first of eight months between parts twelve (17 August 1849)[21] and thirteen (12 April 1850),[22] and one of five months between parts fifteen (1 November 1850)[24] and sixteen (11 April 1851).[25]

A period of eight months intervened before the last two parts[26,27] were published at the end of December 1851. Snow gave no reason for this lengthy delay, but these two articles were separated by an interval of just one week which was not at all typical of the rest of the series. The final article appeared in the last issue of the *London Medical Gazette* before it ceased its separate publication, and such a sequence could hardly have been coincidental. Snow would have been aware for at least four weeks of the *London Medical Gazette*'s impending merger[34] and would have wished to complete the whole series before this led to a change in the journal's format. He was, presumably, encouraged in this by the Editor.

Snow certainly planned to continue his series of articles beyond the sixteenth episode[25] but the last two are not of the same calibre as the earlier ones, and they may have been hurriedly put together against a firm deadline. For some reason, they were indexed in the *London Medical Gazette* in a completely different way from the earlier ones, and a previous study which referred to the work omitted to mention parts seventeen and eighteen altogether.[35]

The slower rate of initial publication of the articles which later comprised the second pamphlet probably reflects the increasing demands which other interests made upon Snow's time, in particular his epidemiological study during and after the cholera outbreak of 1849. This was at its peak in parts of London in July and August of that year, and Snow completed the first, and greatly overlooked, edition of his famous study *On the Mode of Communication of Cholera* at the end of August, 1849. Within a few weeks this work had been published as a pamphlet,[36] but it received a dismissive review in the *London Medical Gazette*.[37] By this time Snow had no doubt, in his own mind, that cholera was a water-borne, infectious disease. However, at the end of his 1849 pamphlet on cholera he had written of his regret that 'being pre-occupied by another subject' (which must have been anaesthesia), he had had no time to round off his study and prove, conclusively, that the disease was spread by infected water. Frustratingly, he had to wait until he had analysed the patterns of London's next great cholera epidemic (in September, 1854) before being able to present sufficient detail to prove his theory and force it into more general acceptance.[2] Quite possibly the disappointing reception, in August 1849, of his work on cholera conditioned Snow's approach to his continuing study of the basic science of anaesthesia. He may well have decided that only an impeccably researched study would be likely to convince those who doubted his progressive opinions on the subject. This would account for the eight month's interval which followed part twelve's publication in the journal in mid-August 1849.[21] When the next instalment[22] eventually appeared Snow ascribed the delay to his wish to repeat many of his experiments, and to perform additional ones (p 65), presumably in order to prove the points he intended to make later in the series.

Snow made many contributions to the literature of medicine, and he did so in a variety of ways for, around the 1840s and 1850s, medical men who wished to promote their views amongst their colleagues had many opportunities for doing so. For example, medical societies flourished throughout most of the country. Those in London ranged from the Royal Medico-Chirurgical Society, the Westminster Medical Society, and the Medical Society of London (at which discussions covered a wide selection of general medical and surgical topics) to specialist societies—such as the

Epidemiological Society of London—which confined their deliberations to narrower fields. Snow made several contributions to each
of these societies' meetings and their proceedings were reported
regularly, and in some detail, in the leading professional journals.
In addition, the journals afforded other opportunities for the
dissemination of knowledge—as articles, or series of articles, either
offered by authors or especially invited by editors, as *verbatim*
accounts of lectures delivered by prominent clinicians, as contributions to the correspondence columns, and (from time to time) in
the course of editorials. In addition, the publication of specialist
textbooks seems to have been relatively commonplace at the time
and, for those with insufficient information or standing to authorise
a textbook, it was remarkably easy to have their own views
published in the form of pamphlets or tracts, of which a plethora
exists.

Although Snow availed himself of each of these methods in order
to promote his views he placed most reliance on the medical
journals, and would have been aware that the early to mid-
nineteenth century had been a period of great development in
medical journalism. Previously, the proceedings or 'house-journals'
of the established scientific and medical societies were considered
to be sufficient. Most were published at a leisurely pace (irregularly,
and quarterly or less often), contained little if anything other than
the relevant society's deliberations and news, and rarely felt it
appropriate to comment upon wider issues or to convey a sense
of urgency about medical matters.

However, in the early to mid-1800s medical advances (both in
the academic and political spheres) began apace, and the need
emerged for periodicals able to handle far more current reporting
than had hitherto been thought either possible or necessary.
Coincidentally, technical achievements (such as improvements
in the technology of printing,[38] the expansion of the railway
system[39] and the advent of the electric telegraph[40]) enabled rapid
communications from centre to centre and over large distances,
and made such a development in journalism possible, as did the
introduction of the 'penny post'.[40] As a result, in 1823, Thomas
Wakley, a far-seeing, opinionated and influential London surgeon,
founded and edited Britain's first weekly medical journal *The
Lancet*.[41] Wakley's purpose was to provide up to the minute
reports and comment on a whole range of medical matters and
politically-relevant events for doctors in London and the provinces.
The Lancet set itself up to monitor the established medical scene,
to encourage progressive thinking amongst doctors, to mould
opinions, and to crusade for improvements. It was successful, and
the pattern for the future of major medical journalism was set. Four
years later, in 1827, the *London Medical Gazette* first appeared,[42]

and this was followed, in 1839, by the *Medical Times*.[43] These three were the principal medical journals of Snow's day. There was intense rivalry between them as each one competed for virtually the same, and relatively small, readership. Eventually in late 1851, the *London Medical Gazette* ceased publication and merged with *The Medical Times*: the combined journal survived until 1885.[44]

Snow was, evidently, widely and well-read, and he contributed to a spectrum of the journals of his day. However, it is difficult to escape the conclusion that, of all the journals with which he was familiar, the *London Medical Gazette* was his favourite. Certainly, the index to this reprinted work shows that it was the journal most often cited during the course of the eighteen essays.

In 1838, within a few months of obtaining his first formal medical qualifications (by which time he had been in London for something less than two years)[45] Snow began to involve himself in wider medical affairs, and also made his first contribution to the medical literature. In December of that year he joined in a debate in the *London Medical Gazette* on the action of the rectus abdominis muscles,[46] giving an independent, robust and reasoned account which conflicted with the views of more established figures.[47] The same volume also recorded that he was a discussant at one of the weekly meetings of the Westminster Medical Society which was held early in January, 1839.[48]

Snow was a member of this society, and thought highly of it (he was later to become its President).[3] Its proceedings, and his own contributions to them, were regularly reported in the *London Medical Gazette*, and elsewhere, in the years before the introduction of anaesthesia. In addition to these Snow made several original contributions to the journal's pages on subjects as diverse as chest and spinal deformities in children[49] and resuscitation of the newborn.[50] He also described an apparatus for paracentesis of the thorax,[51] and gave an account of the capillary circulation.[52] In addition, he wrote letters and case reports. None of the early contributions which Snow made to the journals suggest that he had developed any special interests, or that he was particularly mindful of the, then, medicinal uses of inhalational therapy.

Snow's earliest contributions to anaesthesia demonstrate that he was familiar with many articles which had, earlier, been written by others and published in the *London Medical Gazette*. Indeed, circumstantial evidence indicates that his interest in anaesthesia first came about as a result of his readership of the *London Medical Gazette*, which had been the first British journal to publish the news of anaesthesia's invention in Boston. It did so in its edition dated Friday 18 December 1846,[53] and developed something of a proprietorial interest in the subject during its earliest days.[54]

That same edition also published an original communication from Snow—an illustrated case report of strangulation of the ileum in an aperture of the mesentery.[55] Snow would have been less than human had he not, soon after receiving his copy of the journal, scanned through it to see his case report in print. On thumbing through the rest of the journal his attention must, almost certainly, have been drawn to the enthusiastic annotation entitled 'Animal magnetism superseded—discovery of a new hypnopoietic'.[53]

Within a few days, Snow arranged to visit the premises of the dentist James Robinson (the first man to use anaesthesia in England, and Britain's true pioneer of the subject)[56] and to observe ether anaesthesia for himself. This he did during the morning of Monday 28 December 1846,[57] ten days after this novel use of ether was first mentioned in a British medical journal, and just one week after its first public use in London.[58]

Without delay Snow set about designing an efficient inhaler for ether anaesthesia, and he was readily able to recall a relevant paper which had appeared in a much earlier edition of the *London Medical Gazette*. Several years previously Dr Julius Jeffreys had described an inhaler specifically for warmed air in the treatment of chest disease.[59] Snow based the design of his ether inhaler on Jeffrey's device,[60] and this prototype was in the course of being manufactured within three weeks of his first seeing ether being used.[60] Similarly, in 1851, by which time he had taken a great interest in the use of medicated inhalations and wished to devise an inhaler specifically for giving ammonia,[61] he was able to recall the details of a paper which had appeared in the *London Medical Gazette* in 1843.[62]

(*The Lancet* was the foremost medical journal of the day, and Snow certainly published articles in it but there seems to have been, for some reason, an uneasy relationship between Snow and *The Lancet*. Without citing such unease, it is difficult to explain away the brief, and entirely dismissive, note which appeared in that journal[63] ten days after his death.)

From the very beginning, Snow appreciated that the use of an efficient vapourising device to provide accurate control of vapour strength was essential to the safe and effective practice of anaesthesia. Within a few weeks of its introduction to Britain he was making his views on ether anaesthesia widely known through articles which he wrote for the journals, and in the published reports of medical meetings. A study of the articles on anaesthesia which were written by others around this time shows that the majority were simple or unmeritorious case-reports, pseudo-scientific speculations, and turgid or confusing reviews of the subject. The overall approach was entirely empirical. Virtually alone amongst the earliest anaesthetists Snow appreciated that the subject had a scientific basis which it was important to understand and to apply. Drawing on his own commonsense, his own inquisitiveness of mind, his own practicality, and his own familiarity with the sciences which were to subserve anaesthesia he set out to describe the fundamentals of anaesthetic practice.

In late October 1847 his textbook *On the Inhalation of the Vapour of Ether* was published.[1] It is said that only 126 copies of the work were sold,[64] and Snow may well have been financially disappointed as a result of its limited success at the time. Although his needs were always Spartan he was never rich and, at this stage of his career, this episode may have caused him some concern. Nonetheless, Snow clearly must have considered that he still had a great deal to say about anaesthesia and its safe practice and, equally clearly, he must have been very determined to disseminate his ideas amongst his colleagues. His recent experience of producing a textbook may well have made him wary of repeating the venture, but the publication of a sequence of articles in a reputable journal would have seemed an attractive alternative. It offered Snow the chance, at no particular cost to himself, to reach a prestigious and arguably far wider readership than he had been able to with his textbook on ether.

By the time, in early May 1848, that the *London Medical Gazette* received[65] the first of Snow's series of eighteen articles his reputation as England's foremost anaesthetist was becoming established, as was the process of anaesthesia with both ether and chloroform. Snow had already presented several other communications on the subject, and it is not at all clear what, in particular, prompted him to produce the series of articles at this precise time.

It may, simply, have been an altruistic wish to disseminate his accumulated knowledge on various anaesthetic agents. After chloroform's introduction he had begun to study a whole variety of volatile compounds with a view to establishing their suitability as anaesthetics, and the properties of these agents which related to their anaesthetic potency, safety, and other effects in clinical practice. However, Snow had certainly conceived the idea of writing of chloroform's dangers by February 1848[66] by which time the death of Miss Hannah Greener during a chloroform anaesthetic on Friday 28 January 1848 had been widely reported in the medical and lay journals. A particularly detailed account of the tragedy appeared in the *London Medical Gazette* itself in February 1848,[67] and was followed by considerable discussion in this (and other) journals' columns which continued for some weeks. Snow was entirely dismissive[66] about most of the postulated causes of Hannah Greener's death, and it may have been that the controversy which raged about this unfortunate case (the first fatality attributed confidently to anaesthesia) persuaded him to reflect anew on the unscientific nature of his contemporaries' anaesthetic practice, and of the need for this comprehensive review.

The Editor of the *London Medical Gazette* must have readily appreciated Snow's erudition and growing reputation for he admitted him to the exclusive group of authors who contributed, piecemeal, a lengthy series of specialised articles. The journal, in common with its rivals, published work from several leading authorities in this format, and its readership would have been accustomed to narratives appearing in instalments. Charles Dickens was popular with the educated classes[68] and, at the time, was presenting his current novels (*Dombey and Son*, and *David Copperfield*) in this way.[69]

Snow would have found the arrangement for occasional publication convenient, for it allowed him to devote himself to his other pressing interests as and when he felt it necessary. It would appear that the Editor usually allocated him space in the *London Medical Gazette* whenever he cared to send an instalment along. However, if there was a delay in the publication of his manuscript Snow, it seems, wrote for reassurance that all was well.[70,71]

The erratic timing of the articles' appearance in the journal, coupled with the three and a half year period over which they were published, would have given the Editor of the *London Medical Gazette* many opportunities to curtail Snow's series of essays had he felt that they were failing to maintain their initial momentum or to attract and retain a readership. Quite the reverse may have been the case. In their journal form, the first six articles were not numbered, implying that such a lengthy series was not initially contemplated. However, these early articles were, presumably, satisfactory and it is likely that the Editor suggested, or acceded to the suggestion, that subsequent instalments would be produced as and when Snow had relevant information to impart.

By any yardstick, the calibre of Snow's science displayed in *On Narcotism by the Inhalation of Vapours* is outstanding, and affords a measure of the greatness of the man himself. However, there are several examples within its pages which indicate that Snow was, at times, mistaken in his opinions. These include the significance which he attached to stertor as an indication of anaesthetic depth (pp 23, 45), his speculation on the mechanism by which anaesthetic agents exert their effect (pp 53, 98), his belief that part of this was due to a direct action on peripheral nerves (p 22), and his deductions about anaesthetics and putrefaction (p 96). Given the circumstances of the time it is hardly surprising that Snow was unable to arrive at more satisfactory conclusions on these subjects. The topics themselves, it should be noted, were peripheral to the main thrust of his arguments.

Had he had the benefit of hindsight, the Editor should have felt that his confidence in Snow had been justified, for many of the ideas and concepts formulated in this series of papers were well ahead of their time, and yet were to become fundamental to the efficient use of inhalational anaesthesia. The scope and contents of these articles demonstrate that Snow was a gifted and ingenious researcher. He was readily able to correlate his clinical experience with the results of his laboratory research, both the formal bench-work and animal studies, and his occasional human experiments (usually performed with himself as the subject).

Snow kept careful notes of his clinical practice (both as an anaesthetist and a family doctor) in three manuscript casebooks[72] which, fortunately, still survive. During his extended study of the epidemiology of cholera, and of the two major outbreaks in London in 1849[36] and 1854,[2] he must also have kept extensive and meticulous records although none of these has been preserved. Similarly, in this series of eighteen papers, he recorded details of no less than eighty-three experiments which he had performed, and he referred in passing to a number of others. Snow must have kept records of these experiments for later reference and, indeed, at one point in this work he indicated that he had done so (p 27). Unfortunately, these experimental records no longer exist. Had they survived, they would have afforded even more fascinating detail about his scientific research. Snow had a peripatetic practice, and visited many of London's hospitals without being a full member of their staffs. Presumably, he carried out most of his experiments at his own home in the, then, impoverished Soho district of London.

The pages of this volume abound with examples of Snow's quite extraordinary foresight, and of his real understanding of the scientific foundations of inhalational anaesthesia. Within four years of its introduction, he had enunciated several of the principles on which anaesthetic practice is still based.

His appreciation of the importance of administering an accurate, or controlled strength of vapour during anaesthesia was fundamental to his thinking. Within a matter of days of ether's introduction to Britain Snow declared that an efficient vapouriser was a pre-requisite for safe anaesthesia. He understood the significance of saturated vapour pressure (which he referred to as 'the elastic force' of a vapour (see p 33)), and the experiments which he carried out, for example with ether,[73] to determine how this varied with temperature correspond remarkably accurately with our accepted values.[74] This was no small achievement given the limits of experimental apparatus and method at the time. Based on this work Snow stressed the importance of temperature stability in the design of reliable anaesthetic vapourisers. At the time simple draw-over devices were used and he also emphasised that the resistance which they offered to breathing should be minimal. In addition, these articles show that he understood the concepts which are known today as 'apparatus dead space' and 'anatomical dead space', and was aware of their importance in clinical practice (p 12).

Snow also anticipated the present-day knowledge of pharmaco-kinetics, and his conclusions were amazingly relevant. He conducted his own experiments to determine quantities which would nowadays correspond to blood–gas solubility coefficients. When he came to consider the factors which determined the effects of a whole range of inhalational agents he concluded that the amounts needed to produce anaesthesia were inversely related to their solubilities in blood (p 19). In addition, he assessed the relative potencies of several anaesthetic vapours by calculating the blood levels which would correspond to his various degrees of narcotism (p 61).

When he came to consider the effects of inhalational agents on the body he performed several elegant experiments (pp 81–83) showing how carbon dioxide production diminished during the anaesthetic state and, from these, he deduced the effects which such a state had on 'metabolic rate', although this is a term with which Snow would not have been familiar. He also noted that the fall in body temperature which he observed during some experiments was due to diminished 'oxidation' in the body (p 86). His records of some of his experiments include the first mention, in relation to anaesthesia, of the use of both carbon-dioxide absorption and closed circuit techniques (pp 80, 81).

Snow extended his work on anaesthetics to include studies on the effects of alcohol. He was a strict teetotaller, and these pages contain what appears to be the only surviving account of his personal condemnation of alcohol (p 69). Nonetheless, he recorded in these articles how he, himself, had imbibed alcohol to study its mode of elimination from the body, and to devise a method for its detection in the breath (p 78). Orthodox scientific opinion of the time (set out by Professor Justus von Liebig) decreed that alcohol was not excreted in the breath, and Snow—unabashed by Liebig's pre-eminence as a research chemist—disproved this. Snow was evidently a well-informed and practical chemist. He developed his own series of tests for the detection of chloroform in air, blood and tissues, and went on to make the first anaesthetic contribution to forensic medicine (p 76).

Snow's work, set out in the eighteen papers, was obviously appreciated at the time by the Editor of the *London Medical Gazette*, and the whole collected work attracted an encouraging review in the *London Journal of Medicine* in 1852.[75] However, during Snow's lifetime virtually no other anaesthetist followed his example and seriously investigated the principles underlying anaesthesia.

To all intents and purposes he had, or was given, the monopoly of scientific thought on the subject.

Snow, it seems had a vision of what anaesthesia could, or should, be. That his ideas were not taken up is a paradox which was, almost certainly, a reflection of medical and lay attitudes current during the eleven years or so between anaesthesia's first use, at the end of 1846, and his death in 1858. Prior to late 1846 the opportunity for regular, painless surgery had not existed and the advent of rapid, reversible insensibility induced for operations—simply by the inhalation of ether or chloroform—was perceived as so great an advance that it was almost inconceivable that it could be improved still further. In essence, there had been nothing before and then, unheralded, there was something—and that something answered its purpose very well. The difference between before and after must have seemed infinite. After a few teething troubles anaesthesia had appeared, to most observers, to be reliable and effective. It was yet another example of the ingenuity of man by which life, in this Victorian period of confident advance, was to become more tolerable for all. The occasional deaths which may, or may not, have been associated with its use were too few in number to seriously call the invention into question. Though dramatic, surgery at the time was still a relatively unsophisticated and unscientific practice, and one which carried a fearful mortality rate. There was, it seemed, no great need to put anaesthesia onto a scientific basis: empiricism appeared to be coping well.

With few notable exceptions these attitudes continued for decades after Snow's death. It was well into the twentieth century before anaesthesia was perceived (by a majority of its own practitioners, and others) to be anything more than an ancillary process having at its disposal only three agents, the use of which depended on manual dexterity and experience rather than scientific knowledge.

At a remarkably early stage of anaesthesia's development Snow was uncannily prescient about many, now accepted, aspects of his subject—such as the need for efficient vapourisers and the relevance of saturated vapour pressures ('elastic forces'), the inverse relationship between effect and blood–gas solubility, the use of carbon dioxide absorption and closed circuit techniques, and the assessment of relative potencies of inhalational agents. Yet Boyle, when introducing his machine in 1917, did not incorporate anything resembling an accurate vapouriser.[76] The significance of saturated vapour pressures, the importance of the relationship between anaesthetic effects and blood–gas solubility,[77] the use of carbon dioxide absorption techniques,[78] and the concept of MAC values[79] were not regularly incorporated into anaesthetic thinking until some sixty years, or more, later. When they were introduced little, if any, notice was taken of Snow's pioneering work.

Snow died at the age of forty-five, six and a half years after completing this series of papers for the *London Medical Gazette*. During that time he explored and wrote about many other aspects of anaesthesia. His book on chloroform,[3] published shortly after his death, demonstrated his continued reliance on scientific method and his wish to inform and educate his colleagues. Had he lived longer he would have continued to promote his views about the proper basis of anaesthesia, and would have tried to persuade his contemporaries to adopt his approach. In all probability he would not have succeeded, for Snow was far, far ahead of his time and most of his progressive ideas were, generally, devalued. The medical world acknowledged that his work, on anaesthesia and on cholera, had been useful but scarcely anyone recognised its true worth until many years later.

The note of Snow's death, in *The Lancet*—then the most influential and percipient of all British medical periodicals—is a dispiriting testament to this. It merely said 'This well-known physician died at noon on the 16th. instant, at his home in Sackville Street, from an attack of apoplexy. His researches on chloroform and other anaesthetics were appreciated by the profession'.[63]

The best known account of Snow's life and work is the *Memoir* written by his close friend and colleague, Dr (later Sir) Benjamin Ward Richardson. This was completed within two months of Snow's death and appended to his posthumously-published textbook *On Chloroform and other Anaesthetics*.[3] Richardson's account was written, with Victorian prolixity, at a time when he was twenty-nine years old and still mourning Snow's death. These circumstances require that careful, historical judgement should be exercised when assessing some parts of Richardson's *Memoir*. Nonetheless, it is a most valuable source, and has served as the starting point for most of the subsequent studies of John Snow. In these the impression has often been given that Richardson's *Memoir*, and the three textbooks,[1-3] are the only remaining, or worthy, sources from which information can be gleaned about Snow and his achievements.

Emphatically, this is not so and there is a wealth of his material— albeit largely overlooked—still available for study. It is to be found in the pages of many medical journals, in various other pamphlets, and also in the three-volume set of Snow's manuscript Casebooks[72] in which he recorded his day-to-day activities as both an anaesthetist and a family doctor during the ten years from 1848 until his death. Arrangements are already in hand for the publication of a complete transcription of these unique volumes.

This essay is intended to serve merely as an introduction to Snow's masterly work set out in the accompanying pages. I hope that the republication of *On Narcotism by the Inhalation of Vapours* will stimulate further research, and bring together more of Snow's material from various, disparate sources (of which this facsimile edition is just one). Such studies will be enormously rewarding. They will supplement the account which Richardson left us in his *Memoir*, and enable a new and authoritative picture to emerge of Snow himself, his thinking, his methods, and the environment in which he worked.

RICHARD H ELLIS
February 1991

References

1 Snow, J. *On the Inhalation of the Vapour of Ether in Surgical Operations*. London: Churchill, 1847

2 Snow, J. *On the Mode of Communication of Cholera*. 2nd edn. London: Churchill, 1855

3 Snow, J. *On Chloroform and other Anaesthetics (with a memoir of the author by Benjamin Ward Richardson)*. London: Churchill, 1858

4 Snow, J. *On the Inhalation of the Vapour of Ether in Surgical Operations*. London: Churchill, 1847. [Facsimile edition. Boston: Reproduced with the help of the Boston Medical Library, undated]

5 Snow, J. *On the Inhalation of the Vapour of Ether in Surgical Operations*. London: Churchill, 1847. [Facsimile edition. New York: Wood-Library Museum of Anesthesiology, 1959]

6 Snow, J. *On the Inhalation of the Vapour of Ether in Surgical Operations*. London: Churchill, 1847. [Facsimile edition (Secher, O). Birkerød: Janssenpharma A/S, 1985]

7 Snow, J. *On the Inhalation of the Vapour of Ether in Surgical Operations*. London: Churchill, 1847. [Facsimile edition (Matsuki, A). Tokyo: Iwanami Book Service Center, 1987]

8 Snow, J. *On Chloroform and other Anaesthetics*. London: Churchill, 1858. [Facsimile edition. Chicago: Wood-Library Museum of Anesthesiology, undated]

9 Snow, J. *On the Mode of Communication of Cholera*. 2nd edn. London: Churchill, 1855. [Facsimile edition. New York: The Commonwealth Fund, 1936]

10 Snow, J. On Narcotism by the Inhalation of Vapours, Part 1. *London Medical Gazette* 1848; **6NS**: 850–854

11 Snow, J. On Narcotism by the Inhalation of Vapours, Part 2. *London Medical Gazette* 1848; **6NS**: 893–895

12 Snow, J. On Narcotism by the Inhalation of Vapours, Part 3. *London Medical Gazette* 1848; **6NS**: 1074–1078

13 Snow, J. On Narcotism by the Inhalation of Vapours, Part 4. *London Medical Gazette* 1848; **7NS**: 330–335

14 Snow, J. On Narcotism by the Inhalation of Vapours, Part 5. *London Medical Gazette* 1848; **7NS**: 412–416

15 Snow, J. On Narcotism by the Inhalation of Vapours, Part 6. *London Medical Gazette* 1848; **7NS**: 614–619

16 Snow, J. On Narcotism by the Inhalation of Vapours, Part 7. *London Medical Gazette* 1848; **7NS**: 840–844

17 Snow, J. On Narcotism by the Inhalation of Vapours, Part 8. *London Medical Gazette* 1848; **7NS**: 1020–1025

18 Snow, J. On Narcotism by the Inhalation of Vapours, Part 9. *London Medical Gazette* 1849; **8NS**: 228–235

19 Snow, J. On Narcotism by the Inhalation of Vapours, Part 10. *London Medical Gazette* 1849; **8NS**: 451–456

20 Snow, J. On Narcotism by the Inhalation of Vapours, Part 11. *London Medical Gazette* 1849; **8NS**: 983–985

21 Snow, J. On Narcotism by the Inhalation of Vapours, Part 12. *London Medical Gazette* 1849; **9NS**: 272–277

22 Snow, J. On Narcotism by the Inhalation of Vapours, Part 13. *London Medical Gazette* 1850; **10NS**: 622–627

23 Snow, J. On Narcotism by the Inhalation of Vapours, Part 14. *London Medical Gazette* 1850; **11NS**: 321–327

24 Snow, J. On Narcotism by the Inhalation of Vapours, Part 15. *London Medical Gazette* 1850; **11NS**: 749–754

25 Snow, J. On Narcotism by the Inhalation of Vapours, Part 16. *London Medical Gazette* 1851; **12NS**: 622–627

26 Snow, J. On Narcotism by the Inhalation of Vapours, Part 17. *London Medical Gazette* 1851; **13NS**: 1053–1057

27 Snow, J. On Narcotism by the Inhalation of Vapours, Part 18. *London Medical Gazette* 1851; **13NS**: 1090–1094

28 Snow, J. *On Narcotism by the Inhalation of Vapours. The first seven parts.* London: Privately published, 1848

29 Snow, J. *On Narcotism by the Inhalation of Vapour. Parts eight to sixteen.* London: Privately published, 1851

30 Snow, J. *On Narcotism by the Inhalation of Vapours. Parts XVII and XVIII.* London: Privately published, 1852

31 Snow, John. *British Museum General Catalogue of Printed Books,* Vol 225. London: Trustees of the British Museum, 1964; pp 235–236

32 Snow, John. *Index Catalogue of the Library of the Surgeon-General's Office, United States Army,* Vol. 13. Washington: Government Printing Office, 1892; pp 234–235

33 Snow, John. *The National Union Catalog,* Vol. 553. London: Mansell, 1978; 130

34 Editorial. *London Medical Gazette* 1851; **13NS**: 1103–1104

35 Shephard, DAE. John Snow and Research. *Canadian Journal of Anaesthesia* 1989; **36**: 224–241

36 Snow, J. *On the Mode of Communication of Cholera,* 1st edn. London: Churchill, 1849

37 Review. On the Mode of Communication of Cholera, by John Snow. *London Medical Gazette* 1849; **9NS**: 466–470

38 Printing. *Chamber's Encyclopaedia,* Vol. 8. Philadelphia: Lippincott, 1901; pp 407–415

39 Woodward, EL. *The Age of Reform, 1815–1870.* 1st edn. Oxford: Clarendon Press, 1938

40 Trevelyan, GM. *Illustrated English Social History. Volume 4, The Nineteenth Century.* Harmondsworth: Penguin, 1963

41 *Lancet* 1823; **i**: 1

42 *London Medical Gazette* 1827; **1**: 1

43 *Medical Times* 1839; **1**: 1

44 LeFanu, WR. *British Periodicals of Medicine: a chronological list.* Baltimore: Johns Hopkins Press, 1937

45 Ellis, RH. Dr John Snow. His London residences, and the site for a commemorative plaque in London. In: Boulton, TB and Atkinson, RS, eds. *The History of Anaesthesia. Proceedings of the Second International Symposium on the History of Anaesthesia; July 1987; London.* London: Royal Society of Medicine Services, 1989; pp 1–7

46 Snow, J. Action of recti muscles. *London Medical Gazette* 1839; **23**: 559–560

47 Lonsdale, EF. On the action of the recti muscles of the abdomen. *London Medical Gazette* 1838; **23**: 415–417

48 Annotation. Westminster Medical Society. *London Medical Gazette* 1839; **23**: 619–623

49 Snow, J. On distortions of the chest and spine in children from enlargement of the abdomen. *London Medical Gazette* 1841; **28**: 112–116

50 Snow, J. On asphyxia, and on the resuscitation of still-born children. *London Medical Gazette* 1841; **29**: 222–227

51 Snow, J. On paracentesis of the thorax. *London Medical Gazette* 1842; **29**: 705–707

52 Snow, J. On the circulation in the capillary blood-vessels, and on some of its connections with pathology and therapeutics. *London Medical Gazette* 1843; **31**: 810–816

53 Medical Intelligence. Animal magnetism superseded—discovery of a new hypnopoietic. *London Medical Gazette* 1846; **3NS**: 1085–1086

54 Annotation. Performance of surgical operations during the state of narcotism from ether. *London Medical Gazette* 1847; **4NS**: 38–39

55 Snow, J. Case of strangulation of the ileum in an aperture of the mesentery. *London Medical Gazette* 1846; **3NS**: 1049–1052

56 Ellis, RH. In: Robinson, J. *A Treatise on the Inhalation of the Vapour of Ether.* Facsimile edition. Eastbourne: Baillière Tindall, 1983

57 Robinson, J. Correspondence. *Medical Times* 1847; **15**: 273–274

58 Boott, F. Surgical operations performed during insensibility, produced by the inhalation of sulphuric ether. *Lancet* 1847; **1**: 5–8

59 Jeffreys, J. On artificial climates for the restoration and preservation of health. *London Medical Gazette* 1842; **29**: 814–822

60 Annotation. Westminster Medical Society. *London Medical Gazette* 1847; **4NS**: 156–157

61 Snow, J. On the inhalation of various medicinal substances. *London Journal of Medicine* 1851; **3**: 122–129

62 Smee, A. On the inhalation of ammonia gas as a remedial agent. *London Medical Gazette* 1843; **32**: 59–62

63 Annotation. Dr. John Snow. *Lancet* 1858; **i**: 635

64 Thomas, KB. The Clover/Snow Collection. *Anaesthesia* 1972; **27**: 436–449

65 Annotation. *London Medical Gazette* 1848; **6NS**: 746

66 Snow, J. Remarks on the fatal case of the inhalation of chloroform. *London Medical Gazette* 1848; **6NS**: 277–278

67 Editorial. *London Medical Gazette* 1848; **6NS**: 236–239

68 Holmes, T. *Sir Benjamin Collins Brodie*. London: Fisher Unwin, 1898

69 Dickens, Charles. *Everyman's Encyclopaedia*, Vol. 4. 6th edn. London: Dent, 1978; pp 204–205

70 Notes to Correspondents. *London Medical Gazette* 1850; **10NS**: 528

71 Notes to Correspondents. *London Medical Gazette* 1850; **11NS**: 308

72 Snow, J. *Three Manuscript Volumes of Casebooks* (1848–1858). London: The Royal College of Physicians

73 Snow, J. Table for calculating the strength of ether vapour. *London Medical Gazette* 1847; **4NS**: 219–220

74 Macintosh, RR, Mushin, WW and Epstein, HG. *Physics for the Anaesthetist*, 3rd edn. Oxford: Blackwell, 1963

75 Bibliographical Record. *London Journal of Medicine* 1852; **4**: 154–156

76 Watt, OM. The evolution of the Boyle apparatus, 1917–1967. *Anaesthesia* 1968; **23**: 103–117

77 Kety, SS. The physiological and physical factors governing the uptake of anaesthetic gases by the body. *Anesthesiology* 1950; **11**: 517–526

78 Jackson, DE. New method for production of general analgesia and anesthesia with description of an apparatus used. *Journal of Laboratory and Clinical Medicine* 1915; **1**: 1-12

79 Merkel, G and Eger EI. A comparative study of halothane and halopropane anaesthesia, including a method for determining equipotency. *Anesthesiology* 1963; **24**: 346–357

Pamphlet contents

The first two pamphlets of *On Narcotism by the Inhalation of Vapours* bore their own pages of contents; the third did not. The contents' pages, which appear in this edition, are less detailed than the headings which immediately preceded each of the eighteen instalments published in the *London Medical Gazette*. Some of the headings were omitted when the articles were re-published in pamphlet form. For the sake of completeness the headings are listed below. The pagination refers to this facsimile edition, in which the breaks between successive instalments are not always apparent. The original pages have been enlarged and the whole work has now been indexed.

Contents

Contents

Contents

ON

NARCOTISM

BY THE

INHALATION OF VAPOURS.

BY

JOHN SNOW, M.D.

THE FIRST SEVEN PARTS,

From the London Medical Gazette for 1848.

LONDON

PRINTED BY WILSON AND OGILVY,
57, SKINNER STREET, SNOWHILL.

1848.

CONTENTS.

ON

NARCOTISM

BY THE

INHALATION OF VAPOURS.

———

By JOHN SNOW, M.D.

———

(*From the London Medical Gazette.*)

———

Vapours when inhaled become absorbed. Method of determining the quantity in the blood in different degrees of narcotism. Experiments on animals for this purpose, with chloroform and with ether.

IT is generally admitted that ether and chloroform, when inhaled, are imbibed and enter the blood ; and this has been proved, as regards ether, in more ways than one. That substance has been detected in the blood of animals that have inhaled it ; and I have proved its absorption as follows :—I passed a tame mouse through the quicksilver of a mercurial trough, into a graduated jar containing air and ether vapour, and, after a little time, withdrew it through the mercury, and introduced it, in the same manner, into a jar containing only air. On withdrawing it, and waiting till the air cooled to its former temperature, I found that the mercury had risen considerably in the first jar, and become depressed to some extent in the second ; vapour of ether having been absorbed from one jar, and part of it exhaled into the other.

M. Lassaigne* endeavoured to ascertain the proportion of ether in the blood in etherization, by comparing the tension of the vapour of serum of the blood before and after inhalation, with that of an aqueous solution of ether in certain known proportions. This method would, no doubt, indicate the quantity of ether in the serum at the time it was examined ; but part of the ether would escape from the blood, in the form of vapour, as soon as it came in contact with the air in its exit from the body. He made the quantity of ether in the blood to be 0·0008, or one part in 1250.

Dr. Buchanan*, by considering the quantity of ether expended in inhalation, and making allowance for what is expired, without being absorbed, considered the quantity in the blood of the adult in complete etherization to be not more than half a fluid ounce ; and this is, I believe, a pretty correct estimate.

I consider, however, that I have found a plan of determining more exactly the proportion of ether and of other volatile substances present in the blood in the different degrees of narcotism. It consists in ascertaining the most diluted mixture of vapour and of air that will suffice to produce any particular amount of narcotism ; and is founded on the following considerations, and corroborated by its agreeing with the comparative physiological strength of the various substances.

———

* Comptes Rendus, 8 Mars, 1847 ; and MED. GAZ. vol. xxxix. p. 968.

* MED. GAZ. vol. xxxix. p. 717.

[5]

When air containing vapour is brought in contact with a liquid, as water or serum of blood, absorption of the vapour takes place, and continues till an equilibrium is established ; when the quantity of vapour in both the liquid and air, bears the same relative proportion to the quantity which would be required to saturate them at the temperature and pressure to which they are exposed. If, for instance, the liquid contains one per cent., and would require ten per cent. to saturate it, the air will contain three per cent. if thirty per cent. be the quantity that it could take up. This is only what would be expected to occur ; but I have verified it by numerous experiments in graduated jars over mercury. The intervention of a thin animal membrane may alter the rapidity of absorption, but cannot cause more vapour to be transmitted than the liquid with which it is imbued can dissolve. The temperature of the air in the cells of the lungs and that of the blood circulating over their parietes is the same; and, therefore, when the vapour is too dilute to cause death, and is breathed till no increased effect is produced, the following formula will express the quantity of any substance absorbed :—As the proportion of vapour in the air breathed is to the proportion that the air, or the space occupied by it, would contain if saturated at the temperature of the blood, so is the proportion of vapour absorbed into the blood to the proportion the blood would dissolve.

The plan which I adopted to ascertain the smallest quantity of vapour, in proportion to the air, that would produce a given effect, was to weigh a small quantity of the volatile liquid in a little bottle, and introduce it into a large glass jar covered with a plate of glass ; and having taken care that the resulting vapour was equally diffused through the air, to introduce an animal so small, that the jar would represent a capacious apartment for it, and wait for that period when the effects of the vapour no longer increased.

Experiments with Chloroform.

I will first treat of chloroform, and, passing over a number of tentative experiments, will adduce a few of those which were made after I had ascertained the requisite quantities. The effects produced in these experiments were entirely due to the degree of dilution of the vapour, for the quantity of chloroform employed was, in every instance, more than would have killed the animal in a much shorter time than the experiment lasted if it had been conducted in a smaller jar. It is assumed that the proportions of vapour and air remain unaltered during the experiment, for the quantity absorbed must be limited to what the animal can breathe in the time, which is so small a part of the whole that it may be disregarded.

Exp. 1.—A Guinea pig was placed in a jar, of the capacity of 1600 cubic inches, and the cover being moved a little to one side for a moment, 8 grs. of chloroform were dropped on a piece of blotting paper suspended within. The animal remained in the jar twenty minutes, and was not appreciably affected any part of the time.

Exp. 2.—The same Guinea pig was placed in the same jar, on another occasion, and 12 grs. of chloroform were introduced in the same manner, being three-quarters of a grain for each 100 cubic inches. In about six minutes it seemed drunk. It was allowed to remain for seventeen minutes, but did not become more affected; occasionally it appeared to be asleep, but could be disturbed by moving the jar. On being taken out it staggered, and could not find the way to its cage at first, but it recovered in two or three minutes.

Exp. 3.—Two grains of chloroform were put into a jar containing 200 cubic inches ; it was allowed to evaporate, and the resulting vapour equally diffused by moving the jar ; and then the cover was withdrawn just far enough to introduce a white mouse. After a short time it began to run round continuously in one direction. At the end of a minute it fell down and remained still, excepting a little movement of one or other of its feet now and then. It remained in the same state, and was taken out at the end of five minutes : it flinched on being pinched, tried to walk directly afterwards, and in a minute or so seemed to be completely recovered.

Exp. 4.—A Guinea pig was placed in the jar of 1600 cubic inches' capacity, and 20 grains of chloroform were introduced, as in the two first experiments, being a grain and a quarter for each

100 cubic inches. In two minutes the Guinea pig began to be altered in its manner. At the end of four minutes it was no longer able to stand or walk, but crawled now and then. After seven minutes had elapsed it no longer moved, but lay breathing as in sleep. It was taken out at the end of a quarter of an hour. It moved its limbs as soon as it was touched, flinched on being pinched, and in four minutes was as active as usual.

Exp. 5.—Three grains of chloroform were diffused in the jar of the capacity of 200 cubic inches, and a white mouse introduced. It was not affected at first, but in less than a minute became drowsy, and at the end of a minute appeared insensible, and did not move afterwards. It was allowed to remain two minutes longer; it breathed naturally, and its limbs were not relaxed. When taken out it was insensible to pinching; it began to recover voluntary motion in two minutes.

Exp. 6.—The same mouse was placed in the same jar on the following day, with 3·5 grs., being a grain and three-quarters for each 100 cubic inches. It ran round as before, but fell down in less than a minute, and before the end of the minute ceased to move. It continued breathing in its natural rapid manner till nearly four minutes had expired, when the breathing became very feeble, and immediately afterwards appeared to have ceased. The mouse was taken out just as four minutes had elapsed. It began immediately to give a few deep inspirations at intervals, after which the breathing became natural; it was perfectly insensible to pinching, and did not stir for three minutes. At the end of five minutes it seemed to be recovered, but it did not eat afterwards, and it died on the following day. The state of its organs will be mentioned farther on. The stoppage of respiration and impending death did not seem to be the direct effect of the vapour, but the result of continued and very deep insensibility.

Exp. 7.—A white mouse was placed in the same jar, with 4 grs. of chloroform. At the end of a minute it was lying, but moved its legs for a quarter of a minute longer. When four minutes had elapsed the breathing became slow, and it was taken out. It was totally insensible for the first three minutes after its removal, and recovered during the two following minutes.

Exp. 8.—The same mouse was placed in the same jar on the following day, with 4·5 grs. of chloroform, being 2¼ grs. for each 100 cubic inches. It became more quickly insensible, and at the end of two minutes the breathing was beginning to be affected, when it was taken out. It recovered in the course of five minutes.

Exp. 9.—A white mouse was put into this jar, after 5 grs. of chloroform had been diffused in it, being 2½ grs. to each 100 cubic inches. It was totally insensible in three-quarters of a minute; in a little more than a minute the breathing became difficult, and, before two minutes had expired, the respiration was on the point of ceasing, and it was taken out. The breathing remained difficult for five minutes, but in other five minutes the mouse recovered, and at the end of a quarter of an hour was very active.

It will be remarked that, in these experiments, the mice became much more quickly affected than the Guinea pigs. The reason of this is, their quicker respiration and much more diminutive size. In the last experiment, the quantity of vapour was evidently sufficient to arrest the breathing by its direct influence.

It is evident from the second, third, and fourth of the above experiments, that about one grain of chloroform to each 100 cubic inches of air, suffices to induce the second degree of narcotism, or that state in which the correct relation with the external world is abolished, but in which sensation and ill-directed voluntary movements may exist. Now one grain of chloroform produces 0·767 of a cubic inch of vapour of the sp. gr. 4·2, as given by Dumas; and when it is inhaled, it expands somewhat as it is warmed, from about 60° to the temperature of the body; but it expands only to the same extent as the air with which it is mixed, and therefore the proportions remain unaltered. But air, when saturated with vapour of chloroform at 100°, contains 43·3 cubic inches in 100; and

$$\text{As } 0·767 : 43·3 :: 0·0177 : 1$$

So that if the point of complete saturation be considered as unity, 0·0177, or 1-56th, will express the degree of saturation of the air from which the vapour is immediately absorbed into the blood; and, consequently, also the degree of saturation of the blood itself.

I find that serum of blood at 100°, and at the ordinary pressure of the atmosphere, will dissolve about its own volume of vapour of chloroform; and since chloroform of sp. gr. 1·483 is 288 times as heavy as its own vapour, $0·0177 \div 288$ gives $0·0000614$, or one part in 16,285, as the average proportion of chloroform by measure in the blood, in the second degree of narcotism.

From the fifth experiment it appears that a grain and a half per 100 cubic inches of air is capable of producing the third degree of narcotism; and by the sixth and seventh experiments, it is shewn that from a grain and three-quarters to two grains causes a very complete state of insensibility, which cannot be long continued without danger; but I may remark, that four minutes in a mouse represents a much longer period in the human being, in whom the circulation and respiration are so much less rapid. I think we may take two grains as the average quantity capable of inducing the fourth degree,—the utmost extent of narcotism required, or that can be safely caused in surgical operations; and by the method of calculation above we shall get $0·0354$, or 1-28th, as representing the degree of saturation of the blood, and $0·0001228$ the proportion by measure in the blood.

A greater quantity than this seems to induce the fifth degree of narcotism, embarrassing the respiration; and two and a half grains have the power of directly stopping the respiratory movements. By calculation we obtain $0·0442$, or 1·22nd, as the degree of saturation of the blood which has this effect.

Birds have generally a somewhat higher temperature than most mammalia, and therefore the following five experiments have been separated from the rest; but, in 13 and 14, the thermometer placed under the wing of the linnet, at the end of the experiment, indicated only 100°,—just the temperature in the groin of the Guinea pig when it was removed from the jar in the 4th experiment. These are the only occasions on which it occurred to me to apply the thermometer.

Exp. 10.—4·6 grs. of chloroform were put into a jar containing 920 cubic inches, by sliding the glass which covered it a little to one side. The jar was moved about to diffuse the vapour; and thus each 100 cubic inches of air contained half a grain. A hen chaffinch was introduced, by again momentarily sliding the cover a little to one side. In less than two minutes it seemed rather unsteady in its walking at the bottom of the jar, but no further effect was produced, although it remained twenty minutes; when taken out, indeed, it did not seem affected. This experiment was repeated on the same bird, and on another chaffinch, and also on a green linnet, with the same result; that is, no decided effect was produced.

Exp. 11.—9·2 grs. of chloroform were diffused through the air in the same jar, being one grain to each 100 cubic inches; and a chaffinch was put in. In less than two minutes it staggered about, and in two and a half minutes fell down, but still stirred. It did not get further affected, although it remained ten minutes. Sometimes it seemed perfectly insensible, but always stirred when the jar was moved, and occasionally it made voluntary efforts to stand. On being taken out it seemed sensible of its removal; it flinched on being pinched, and quickly recovered.

Exp. 12.—A chaffinch was placed in the same jar with 11·5 grs., being a grain and a quarter for each 100 cubic inches. In less than a minute it began to stagger, and shortly afterwards was unable to stand, but moved its legs and opened its eyes occasionally. It did not get further affected after two minutes had elapsed, although it remained three minutes longer. It seemed aware of its removal, but was not sensible to being pricked. In attempting to walk when placed on the table, immediately after its removal from the vapour, it fell forwards at every two or three steps. In a minute or two, however, it was able to walk.

Exp. 13.—A green linnet was put in the same jar, with 13·8 grs., being a grain and a half to each 100 cubic inches. In a minute it was unable to stand, and in half a minute more ceased to move. It remained breathing naturally, and kept its eyes open. It was taken out at the end of ten minutes, was insensible to having its foot pinched, and began to recover voluntary motion in three minutes.

Exp. 14—Was performed on the same linnet, two or three days before the last, with a grain and three-quarters of chloroform to each 100 cubic inches, in the same jar. It was affected much in the same way as detailed above, but was longer in recovering voluntary motion after its removal, at the end of ten minutes.

It will be perceived that these results coincide as nearly as possible with the effects of the same quantities on the Guinea pigs and mice; and I found that when the quantity of chloroform exceeded two grains to the 100 cubic inches, birds were killed very rapidly.

It occurred to me that if this method of ascertaining the amount of vapour in the blood were correct, then a much more dilute vapour ought to suffice to produce insensibility in animals of cold blood; and that experimenting on them would completely confirm or invalidate these views.

The following experiment has been performed on frogs several times with the same result, the temperature of the room being about 55°.

Exp. 15.—4·6 grs. of chloroform were diffused through the jar of 920 cubic inches capacity, as in Exp. 10. In the course of a few minutes the frog began to be affected, and at the end of ten minutes was quite motionless and flaccid; but the respiration was still going on. Being now taken out, it was found to be insensible to pricking, but recovered in a quarter of an hour. In a repetition of this experiment, in which the frog continued a few minutes longer, the respiration also ceased, and the recovery was more tardy. On one occasion the frog was left in the jar for an hour, but when taken out and turned over, the pulsations of the heart could be seen. In an hour after its removal it was found to be completely recovered.

Now the vapour is absorbed into the blood of the frog at the temperature of the external air, whose point of saturation, therefore, remains unaltered; and as half a grain of chloroform produces 0·383 cubic inches of vapour; and air at 55° will contain, when saturated, 10 per cent. of vapour; 0·0383, or 1-26th, expresses the degree of saturation of the air, and also of the blood of the frog. And this is a little more

than 0·0354, or 1-28th, which we considered as the greatest quantity that could with safety exist in the blood. But frogs are able to live without pulmonary respiration, by means of the action of the air on the skin: consequently this experiment coincides exactly with the others, and remarkably confirms the accuracy of this method of determining the amount of chloroform in the blood.

At the College of Physicians, on March 29, when I had the honour of shewing the effects of chloroform at Dr. Wilson's Lumleian Lectures, and briefly explained these views, I conjoined the last experiment and the 10th in the following manner. I introduced a chaffinch, in a very small cage, into a glass jar holding nearly 1000 cubic inches, and put a frog into the same jar, covered it with a piece of glass, and dropped 5 grs. of chloroform on a piece of blotting paper suspended within. In less than ten minutes the frog was insensible, but the bird was unaffected. Then, in order to shew that the effects depended entirely on the dilution of the vapour, another frog, and another small bird, were placed in a jar containing but 200 cubic inches, with exactly the same quantity of chloroform. In about a minute and a half they were both taken out,—the bird totally insensible, but the frog not appreciably affected, as from its less active respiration it had not had time to absorb much of the vapour.

As the narcotism of frogs, by vapour too much diluted to affect animals of warm blood, depends merely on their temperature, it follows that, by warming them, they ought to be put into the same condition, in this respect, as the higher classes of animals; and although I have not raised their temperature to the same degree, I have found that as it is increased, they cease to be affected by dilute vapour that would narcotise them at a lower temperature.

Exp. 16.—I placed the jar holding 920 cubic inches near the fire, with a frog and a thermometer in it; and when the air within reached 75°, 4·6 grains of chloroform were diffused through it. The jar was kept for twenty minutes, with the thermometer indicating the same temperature within one degree. For the first seventeen minutes the frog was unaffected, and only was dull and sluggish, but not insensible when taken out.

Experiments with Ether.

We will now proceed to consider ether, and will begin with the brief relation of a few experiments, shewing the strength of its vapour required to produce narcotism to various degrees.

Exp. 17.—Two grains of ether were put into a jar holding 200 cubic inches, and the vapour diffused equally, when a tame mouse was introduced, and allowed to remain a quarter of an hour, but it was not appreciably affected.

Exp. 18.—Another mouse was placed in the same jar, with three grains of ether, being a grain and a half to each 100 cubic inches. In a minute and a half it was unable to stand, but continued to move its limbs occasionally. It remained eight minutes without becoming further affected. When taken out it was sensible to pinching, but fell over on its side in attempting to walk. In a minute and a half the effect of the ether appeared to have gone off entirely.

Exp. 19.—A white mouse in the same jar, with four grains of ether, was unable to stand at the end of a minute, and at the end of another minute ceased to move, but continued to breathe naturally, and was taken out at the end of five minutes. It moved on being pinched, began to attempt to walk at the end of a minute, and in two minutes more seemed quite recovered.

Exp. 20.—Five grains of ether, being two and a half grains to each 100 cubic inches, were diffused throughout the same jar, and a mouse put in. It became rather more quickly insensible than the one in the last experiment. It was allowed to remain eight minutes. It moved its foot a very little when pinched, and recovered in the course of four minutes.

Exp. 21.—A white mouse was placed in the same jar with six grains of ether. In a minute and a half it was lying insensible. At the end of three minutes the breathing became laborious, and accompanied by a kind of stertor. It continued in this state till taken out, at the end of seven minutes, when it was found to be totally insensible to pinching. The breathing improved at the end of a minute; it began to move

at the end of three minutes; and five minutes after its removal it had recovered.

Exp. 22.—The same mouse was put into this jar on the following day, with seven grains of ether, being 3·5 grs. to the 100 cubic inches. Stertorous breathing came on sooner than before; it seemed at the point of death when four minutes had elapsed; and being then taken out, was longer in recovering than after the last experiment.

Exp. 23.—Two or three days afterwards the same mouse was placed in the jar, with eight grains of ether, being four grains for each 100 cubic inches. It became insensible in half a minute. In two minutes and a half the breathing became difficult, and at a little more than three minutes it appeared that the breathing was about to cease, and the mouse was taken out. In a minute or two the breathing improved, and in the course of five minutes from its removal it had recovered.

The temperature of the mice employed in the above experiments was about 100°. That of the birds in the following experiments was higher, as is stated; and they differ widely from the mice in the strength of vapour required to produce a given effect, although I found but little difference between the mice and birds, in this respect, in the former experiments on chloroform. And one of the linnets was employed in both sets of experiments. Having seen MM. Dumeril and Demarquay's statement of the diminution of animal temperature from inhalation of ether and chloroform, before the following experiments were performed, the thermometer was applied at the beginning and conclusion of some of them. I have selected every fourth experiment from a larger series on birds.

Exp. 24.—18·4 grs. of ether were diffused through a jar holding 920 cubic inches, being two grains to each 100 cubic inches; and a green linnet was introduced. After two or three minutes it staggered somewhat, and in a few minutes more appeared so drowsy, that it had a difficulty in holding up its head. It was taken out at the end of a quarter of an hour, quite sensible, and in a minute or two was able to get on its perch. The temperature under the wing was 110° before the experiment began, and the same at the conclusion.

Exp. 25.—Another linnet was placed in the same jar, with four grains of ether to each 100 cubic inches of air. In two minutes it was unable to stand, and in a minute more voluntary motion had ceased. It lay breathing quietly till taken out, at the end of a quarter of an hour. It moved its foot slightly when it was pinched. In three minutes it began to recover voluntary motion, and was soon well. The temperature was 110° under the wing, when put into the jar, and 105° when taken out.

Exp. 26.—A green linnet was put into the same jar with 55·2 grs. of ether, being six grains to the 100 cubic inches. It was insensible in a minute and a half, and lay motionless, breathing naturally, till taken out at the end of a quarter of an hour. It moved its toes very slightly when they were pinched with the forceps, and it began to recover voluntary motion in two or three minutes. Temperature 110° before the experiment, and 102° at the end.

Exp. 27.—A linnet was placed in the same jar, containing eight grains of ether to each 100 cubic inches. Voluntary motion ceased at the end of a minute. The breathing was natural for some time, but afterwards became feeble, and at the end of four minutes appeared to have ceased; and the bird was taken out, when it was found to be breathing very gently. It was totally insensible to pinching. The breathing improved, and it recovered in four minutes.

Exp. 28.—9·2 grs. of ether, being one grain to each 100 cubic inches of air, were diffused through the jar holding 920 cubic inches of air, and a frog was introduced. At the end of a quarter of an hour it had ceased to move spontaneously, but could be made to move its limbs, by inclining the jar so as to turn it over. At the end of half an hour voluntary motion could no longer be excited, and the breathing was slow. It was removed at the end of three-quarters of an hour, quite insensible, and the respiratory movements being performed only at long intervals, but the heart beating naturally; and it recovered in the course of half an hour. The temperature of the room was 55° at the time of this experiment.

We find from the 18th experiment, that a grain and a half of ether for each 100 cubic inches of air, is sufficient to induce the second degree of narcotism in the mouse; and a grain and a half of ether make 1·9 cubic inches of vapour, of sp. gr. 2·586. Now the ether I employed boiled at 96°. At this temperature, consequently, its vapour would exclude the air entirely; and ether vapour in contact with the liquid giving it off, could only be raised to 100° by such a pressure as would cause the boiling point of the ether to rise to that temperature. That pressure would be equal to 32·4 inches of mercury, or 2·4 inches above the usual barometrical pressure; and the vapour would be condensed somewhat, so that the space of 100 cubic inches would contain what would be equivalent to 108 cubic inches at the usual pressure. This is the quantity, then, with which we have to compare 1·9 cubic inches, in order to ascertain the degree of saturation of the space in the air-cells of the lungs, and also of the blood; and by calculation, as when treating of chloroform,

$$1·9 \text{ is to } 108 \text{ as } 0·0175 \text{ is to } 1.$$

So that we find 0·0175, or 1-57th, to be the amount of saturation of the blood by ether necessary to produce the second degree of narcotism; and as by Exp. 21, three grains in 100 cubic inches produced the fourth degree of narcotism, we get 0·035, or 1-28th, as the amount of saturation of the blood in this degree. Now this is within the smallest fraction of what was found to be the extent of saturation of the blood by chloroform, requisite to produce narcotism to the same degrees. But the respective amount of the two medicines in the blood differs widely; for whilst chloroform required about 288 parts of serum to dissolve it, I find that 100 parts of serum dissolve 5 parts of ether at 100°; consequently 0·05 × 0·0175 gives 0·000875, or one part in 1142, as the proportion in the blood in the second degree of narcotism, and 0·05 × 0·035 gives 0·00175, or one part in 572, as the proportion in the fourth degree.

In Exp. 28, the frog was rendered completely insensible by vapour of a strength which was not sufficient to produce any appreciable effect on the mouse in Exp. 17. This is in accordance with what was met with in the experiments with chloroform. Air, when saturated with ether at 55°, contains 32 grains ; so that the blood of the frog might contain 1-32d part as much as it would dissolve, which, although not quite so great a proportion as was considered the average for the fourth degree in the mice, yet was more than sufficient to render insensible the mouse in Exp. 20.

There is a remarkable difference between the birds and the mice in respect to the proportions of ether and air required to render them insensible, a difference that was not observed with respect to chloroform. In some experiments with ether on Guinea pigs, which are not adduced, they were found to agree with mice in the effects of various quantities.

The birds were found to require nearly twice as much : five grains to 100 cubic inches, the quantity used in an experiment between the 25th and 26th, which is not related, may be taken as the average for the fourth degree of narcotism in these birds, with a temperature of 110°. By the kind of calculation made before, we should get a higher amount of saturation of the blood than for the same degree in the mice. But as serum at 110° dissolves much less ether than at 100°, the quantity of this medicine in the blood of birds is not greater than in that of other animals ; and considered in relation to what the blood would dissolve at 100°, the degree of saturation is the same.

By Expts. 22, 23, and 27, we find that with ether as with chloroform, a quantity of vapour in the air somewhat greater than suffices to induce complete narcotism has the effect of arresting the respiratory movements. The exact amount which has this effect might be determined if necessary.

Before proceeding to consider some other vapours, and the general conclusions to be drawn from these inquiries, it may be as well to consider how far the above results coincide with experience as to the quantities of chloroform and ether required to produce insensibility in the human subject.

The blood in the human adult is calculated by M. Valentin to average about 30 pounds. This quantity would contain 26 pounds five ounces of serum, which, allowing for its specific gravity, would measure 410 fluid ounces. This being reduced to minims, and multiplied by 0·0000614, the proportion of chloroform in the blood required to produce narcotism to the second degree, gives 12 minims as the whole quantity in the blood. And to produce narcotism to the fourth degree we should have twice as much, or 24 minims. More than this is used in practice, because a considerable portion is not absorbed, being thrown out again when it has proceeded no further than the trachea, the mouth and nostrils, or even the face-piece. But I find that if I put twelve minims into a bladder containing a little air, and breathe it over and over again, in the manner of taking nitrous oxide, it suffices to remove consciousness, producing the second degree of its effects.

In order to find the whole quantity of ether in the blood, we may multiply 410, the number of fluid ounces of serum, by 0·000875 for the second degree, and by 0·00175 for the fourth degree, when we shall obtain 0·358 and 0·71 of an ounce, i. e. f$\mathfrak{z}$ij. $\mathfrak{m}$l. in the first instance, and f$\mathfrak{z}$v. $\mathfrak{m}$xl. in the second,—quantities which agree very well with experience when we allow for what is expired without being absorbed.

Experiments to determine the quantity in the blood, and illustrate the action of nitric ether, bisulphuret of carbon, and benzin.

Nitric ether, or nitrate of the oxide of ethyle, consists of nitric acid combined with ordinary or sulphuric ether. It is described as a colourless liquid of sp. gr. 1·112, with a sweet taste and pleasant smell, and boiling at 185° Fah. Two specimens of it which I have answer to this description. One was made and presented to me by Mr. Bullock; and the other, which was made by Mr. Joseph Spence, was given to me by Dr. Barnes. Dr. Chambert, of Paris, related some experiments that he had performed on dogs with the vapour of this substance, in a work on Ether, published in autumn last; and Dr. Simpson afterwards mentioned it in his pamphlet on Chloroform, as one of the things that he had tried.

The two following experiments will serve to determine the quantity of nitric ether in the blood, when insensibility is induced by it:—

EXP. 29.—Four grains were diffused through the air in a jar containing 800 cubic inches; and a common mouse was introduced in the same manner as in the preceding experiments. In ten minutes it became rather torpid, but could be disturbed by touching the jar. It was left in this condition when it had been in a quarter of an hour. On returning at the end of an hour from the commencement of the experiment, I found the mouse lying still. It was taken out, and it moved spontaneously, endeavouring to walk, but falling over; it was quite sensible to being pinched. In five minutes it had recovered power to walk, but was not yet conscious of danger, as it would have walked off the table if not prevented. In a few minutes longer it had recovered its usual state.

EXP. 30.—Another mouse was placed in the same jar with eight grs. of nitric ether. It became affected in ten minutes, and at the end of a quarter of an hour had ceased to move, but lay breathing naturally 160 times in the minute. It remained in this state till removed half an hour after the commencement of the experiment, when it was found to be relaxed, and totally insensible. It began to move in ten minutes; it could walk at the end of a quarter of an hour, and in a little time longer was quite active.

We perceive from the above experiments that half a grain of nitric ether to each 100 cubic inches of air suffices to induce the second degree of narcotism, and one grain the fourth degree. I have not met with a statement of the specific gravity of the vapour of this ether in any work to which I have referred, and consequently I endeavoured to determine it myself—not with great nicety, but with sufficient accuracy to satisfy the purpose of this inquiry. I made it to be 5·67; and half a grain of vapour of this specific gravity will be found on calculation to occupy 0·284 of a cubic inch. The quantity of this vapour in 100 cubic inches of air saturated with it at 100°, is 15·7 cubic inches, and 0·284÷15·7 will give 0·018, or rather less than one fifty-fifth, as the relative saturation of the blood with nitric ether in the second degree of narcotism. One grain produces 0·568 of a cubic inch of vapour: and this, divided by 15·7, gives 0·0361, or very nearly one twenty-eighth, as the relative saturation of the blood in the fourth degree of narcotism. So we find that the quantity of the vapour in the blood, viewed in relation to what it would dissolve, is the same as in the cases of chloroform and sulphuric ether. In some experiments on birds, a rather larger quantity of vapour was required; but when their higher temperature was taken into account the relative proportion to what the air would take up was found to be the same, and, consequently, their blood was saturated to just the same extent.

One part by measure of nitric ether requires 52 parts of serum at 100° to dissolve it, and 52×56=2912; consequently, one part in 2912 is the proportion in the blood in the second degree of narcotism; and considering the average quantity of serum in the body, as before, to be 410 fluidounces, we get by calculation 67 minims as the whole quantity in the blood in this degree; and twice as much, or 2 drachms and 14 minims, in the fourth degree. These quantities agree with the little experience I have had of its effects on the human subject.

From its slight pungency, and the gradual way in which, owing to its sparing volatility, its effects are pro-

c

duced, nitric ether would be a very safe anæsthetic, suitable for minor surgical operations if its effects were agreeable, but such is apparently not always the case. M. Chambert met with vomiting in most of the dogs to which he gave it, and was deterred from inhaling it himself. Dr. Simpson states, in the Monthly Journal of April last, that he had found it to produce sensations of noise and fulness in the head before insensibility, and, usually, much headache and giddiness afterwards. I have inhaled a small quantity of it on two or three occasions, and it caused a disagreeable feeling of sickness each time. I have given it only to one patient, but in that instance it acted very favourably. A middle-aged man applied at St. George's Hospital, on May 26, to have a tooth extracted. He inhaled from the apparatus I use for chloroform. Soon after he began his pulse became accelerated and increased in force, and his face rather flushed. He continued to inhale steadily for three minutes, when I found that the sensibility of the conjunctiva was considerably diminished, although voluntary motion continued in the eyes and eyelids, the expression of his countenance not being altered from that of complete consciousness; and he held his head upright. The vapour was left off, and the tooth, which was firmly fixed, was taken out by Mr. Price, the dresser for the week, without any sign of the operation being felt; the man holding his mouth wide open in an accommodating manner. A minute afterwards he began to spit on the floor; and being questioned, he said that he had no knowledge of the removal of the tooth, and should have thought that he had never lost his senses, except for what he found had been done. His feelings were not unpleasant whilst inhaling, and he felt well, and walked away in a few minutes afterwards. A fluid-drachm and a half was employed, and it was not all used. There was perfect immunity from pain, whilst the narcotism of the nervous centres was not carried further than the second degree: this, however, I do not look on as a peculiarity of nitric ether, for I have met with it occasionally from chloroform and sulphuric ether when the vapour was introduced slowly. The above case, I think, affords encouragement for further trials of this medicine.

Bisulphuret of Carbon.

This substance is well known to every one at all conversant with chemistry. It is a transparent colourless liquid, of sp. gr. 1·272, having a very fœtid odour, and boiling at about 113°. A paragraph copied from the Morgenblad went the round of the journals of this country about the end of February last, stating that M. Harald Thanlow, of Christiana, in Norway, had discovered a substitute for chloroform and ether, in a sulphate of carbon, a very cheap substance made from sulphur and charcoal. This, of course, could be nothing else than the bisulphuret of carbon. I immediately examined its effects on animals, and found that it causes convulsive tremors, but that the kind of narcotism such as ether produces may be recognised. On account of the great volatility and very sparing solubility of this substance, the point of relative saturation of the blood by it is soon reached.

The following experiments will shew both the action of the vapour and the quantity of it in the blood.

EXP. 31.—Two grains of bisulphuret of carbon were diffused through the air in a jar holding 200 cubic inches, and a white mouse was introduced. In three minutes it was altered in its manner, and no longer regarded the approach of the hand towards it. In six minutes tremors came on, which soon became violent, and lasted till after the mouse was taken out at the end of ten minutes; but voluntary motion continued along with the tremors. When taken out, it flinched on being pinched; attempted to walk, but fell over on its side: it had no appreciation of danger at first, but it quickly recovered.

EXP. 32.—A common mouse was put into a jar holding 800 cubic inches, in which 12 grains of bisulphuret of carbon had been diffused, being a grain and a half to each 100 cubic inches. In a minute it began to have convulsive tremors whilst still walking. In half a minute more, voluntary motion ceased, but the tremors continued. It was removed at the end of ten minutes, was sensible to pricking and pinching, and in a minute or two began to recover voluntary motion, the trembling of the whole body continuing for a little time after it was able to walk.

Exp. 33.—A white mouse was placed in the jar of 200 cubic inches capacity, with four grains of this substance in the form of vapour. It became quickly affected, and was lying powerless in less than half a minute. Convulsive tremors came on immediately after it fell, and lasted till death. At the end of four minutes the breathing became difficult, being performed only by distant convulsive efforts. The mouse was immediately removed, but only gave one or two gasps afterwards.

In another experiment, in which there were two and a quarter grains to each 100 cubic inches of air, the mouse, after running about for a minute, fell down, and stretched itself violently out, and died.

There is no stage of muscular relaxation prior to death by this vapour, as by those we have previously considered, when their effects are gradually induced; but tremulous convulsions of the whole body continue till death, which seems to be threatened almost as soon as complete insensibility to external impressions is established.

In Exp. 31, narcotism to the second degree was occasioned by one grain to 100 cubic inches. The sp. gr. of the vapour of bisulphuret of carbon being 2·668, it will be found that one grain of the liquid must produce 1·209 cubic inches of vapour; and I find that air, when saturated with it at 100°, expands to four times its former volume, so that 100 cubic inches contain 75 of vapour. Therefore 1·209÷75 gives 0·0161, or one part in 62 of what the blood would dissolve, as the relative saturation of the blood in the second degree of narcotism; and, as Exp. 33 may be regarded as the nearest approach to the fourth degree that we can get with this vapour, twice as much, or one part in 31, is the relative amount for that degree. These proportions do not differ much from those arrived at in the inquiries concerning the vapours previously examined.

Serum at 100° dissolves, as nearly as I can determine, just its own volume of the vapour of bisulphuret of carbon; and, as the liquid is 408 times as heavy as its own vapour at the temperature of 100°, it will be found, by a similar calculation to that made with respect to the vapours treated of previously, that about 7½ minims is the average quantity that there should be in the whole blood of the human subject in the second degree, and 15 minims in the fourth degree of narcotism. When the great volatility of this substance is also taken into account, it will be perceived that its effects, when inhaled, must be most powerful. Indeed, I feel convinced, that, if a person were to draw a single deep inspiration of air, saturated with its vapour at a summer temperature, instant death would be the result. Although its odour is offensive, it is not difficult to inhale; and Dr. Simpson has given it in a surgical operation and an obstetric case; he also informs us (op. cit.) that its effects were so powerful and so transient, that it was very unmanageable, and that it also caused some unpleasant symptoms, and he does not recommend its use.

Benzin or Benzole.

This substance was first discovered by Dr. Faraday, as a product of the distillation of compressed oil-gas, and named bicarburet of hydrogen; it was afterwards obtained by Mitscherlich, by distilling a mixture of benzoic acid and slaked lime; latterly Mr. Blatchford Mansfield has obtained it by the distillation of coal-tar. It consists of carbon and hydrogen, as its first name implied, the proportions being $C_{12}H_6$. It is a clear, colourless, and very mobile liquid, of sp. gr. 0·85, and having an aromatic odour. It has been described as boiling at 186°, but some which Mr. Bullock made from benzoic acid, and carefully rectified, boiled at 180°; and a portion with which Mr. Mansfield favoured me, boils, as he always found it to do, about 178°. There is no difference either in sensible properties or physiological effects between the benzin made from benzoic acid, and that obtained from coal-tar. Like the substance last treated of, it causes convulsive tremors in addition to the other symptoms of narcotism; they usually begin in animals before voluntary motion ceases, and continue as long as the vapour is applied, and during part of the recovery, and until death when animals are killed by it. The tremors are usually violent, affecting the whole body, and accompanied in birds with flapping of the wings.

One experiment will suffice to shew the effects of this vapour.

Exp. 34.—Six grains of benzin were diffused through the air in a jar holding 800 cubic inches, being three-quarters of a grain for each 100 cubic inches; and a half-grown white mouse was introduced. In less than a minute it began to shake and tremble, and ceased to move voluntarily, but every now and then gave a sudden start; this start could also be occasioned at any time by striking the jar so as to make a noise. This mouse continued in the same state till removed at the end of a quarter of an hour; it was totally insensible to pricking and pinching, which produced not the slightest effect on it, whilst at the same time a sharp noise near it caused it to start. Five minutes after its removal it began to recover voluntary motion, but the tremors continued a little longer. The mouse was soon as well as before the experiment. Less than half a grain of benzin to each 100 cubic inches of air, suffices to impair the voluntary motion, and alter the manner of an animal; rather more than half a grain causes convulsive tremors, and three-quarters of a grain and upwards produces complete insensibility, whilst two grains will take away life. In the experiment related above, the fourth degree of narcotism appeared to be induced by three-quarters of a grain, but one grain to the 100 cubic inches of air is the average quantity for that stage in several experiments. The specific gravity of the vapour of benzin being 2·738, one grain of the liquid makes 1·179 cubic inch of vapour; and I find that air saturated with it at 100°, contains 20 per cent. of it by measure: so $1·179 \div 20$ will give the relative saturation of the blood. It is 0·058, or one-seventeenth part of what it would dissolve. This is a greater proportion than we arrived at in examining the vapours treated of above.

Benzin requires 270 parts of serum for its solution; consequently, by the kind of calculation made before, 42 minims is obtained as the average quantity that there would be in the human body, if narcotism were carried to the fourth degree by this vapour. It follows from this that benzin must be powerful in its effects, and such I have found to be the case, but they are not so rapidly produced as the effects of chloroform, on account of its lesser volatility. I employed it in some cases of tooth-drawing, and in one amputation, in St. George's Hospital, at the latter part of last year. Its action in the minor operations was very

nearly the same as that of nitric ether, in the case related above; but in the amputation, where its effects were carried further, the patient had violent convulsive tremors for about a minute, which, although not followed by any ill consequences, were sufficiently disagreeable to deter me from using it again, or recommending it in the larger operations.

Bromoform.

This is a volatile liquid of the same composition as chloroform, except that three atoms of bromine occupy the place of the same proportion of chlorine. It is made in the same way as chloroform, bromide of lime being used instead of chloride. I have repeatedly made it, but have never succeeded in obtaining more than a few grains in a purified state, although I used an ounce of bromine in making the bromide of lime on each occasion; consequently it is very expensive. It is extremely fragrant, having an odour that is, in my opinion, much pleasanter than that of chloroform or any other of this class of substances with which I am acquainted. It boils at about 184° Fah.; but, as its vapour is twice as heavy as that of chloroform, it is in point of fact nearly as volatile as that liquid. It is very pleasant to inhale, but I have never breathed more than a few grains at a time, and, therefore, cannot speak of its operation on the human subject. Its effects on animals closely resemble those of chloroform.

The two following experiments will serve to illustrate the action of bromoform, and to determine the quantity in the blood:—

EXP. 35.—A common mouse was placed in a jar containing 400 cubic inches, in which three grains of bromoform had been diffused. In the course of four or five miuntes it became unsteady in its walking, and ceased to regard objects in its way. It did not get further affected, except to become rather sluggish, and, when removed at the end of twenty minutes, was capable of voluntary motion. It did not regard a slight pinch, but flinched when the soft part of its foot was pinched severely. It recovered gradually, and was pretty well re-established in half an hour.

EXP. 36.—Another mouse was placed in the same jar with six grains of bromoform: it was more quickly affected, and, at the end of five minutes, all voluntary motion had ceased, and it lay breathing naturally and rather deeply. It was removed at the end of a quarter of an hour, and did not stir on being pinched. It began to recover voluntary motion in ten minutes, but staggered at first. In a little more than half an hour it had recovered.

In the first of these experiments the second degree of narcotism was caused by three-quarters of a grain of bromoform to each 100 cubic inches of air. The specific gravity of the vapour of bromoform is stated, in Thompson's Chemistry of Organic Bodies, to be 8·785, which gives 0·275 of a cubic inch as the quantity of vapour that three-quarters of a grain would yield; and I find that fifteen cubic inches of this vapour are contained in 100 of air saturated with it at the temperature of 100°; consequently the air of the jar contained $0·275 \div 15 = 0·0183$, or nearly one fifty-fourth part of what it would take up if saturated at 100°, and, according to the principles explained in a former part of these papers,* the blood of the mouse would contain just the same proportion—one fifty-fourth of what it could dissolve. In the other experiment, the fourth degree of narcotism was produced by twice the quantity—a grain and a half to each 100 cubic inches, which, by the same computation, gives about one twenty-seventh part of what the blood would take up. These proportions are nearly the same as in the case of most of the substances previously examined. I have not ascertained the exact solubility of bromoform, and consequently cannot compute the absolute quantity in the blood, but it resembles chloroform in being very sparingly soluble.

I have not heard that any one else has examined the effects of the vapour of bromoform; but Dr. Glover mentions an experiment in his valuable paper On Bromine and its Compounds,† in which bromoform in the liquid state was introduced into the stomach of a rabbit, with the same results as in other experiments with similar bodies: these were death, with congestion of the lungs and stomach.

Bromide of Ethyle.

Bromide of ethyle, or hydrobromic

ether, is a very volatile liquid, boiling, as I have found, at 104°. It has a pleasant but somewhat pungent taste and smell. It was discovered by Serullas in 1827, and is formed by the action of phosphorus on a solution of bromine in alcohol. I am not aware that its physiological effects have been examined except in a few experiments which I have performed with its vapour. I will cite two of them to illustrate its effects. The bromide of ethyle was made by myself.

Exp. 37.—Eight grains of bromide of ethyle were introduced into a jar containing 400 cubic inches, and the vapour which instantly resulted was equally diffused by moving the jar. A mouse was then put in. In about four minutes it began to stagger and fall over, and was quite regardless of external objects. It did not get affected beyond this extent, except that it became rather feeble. It was taken out at the end of a quarter of an hour, having the power of voluntary motion, but rolling over in its attempts to walk. It flinched with severe, but not with slight pinching. In ten minutes it had pretty well recovered.

Exp. 38.—Another mouse was placed in the same jar with sixteen grains of bromide of ethyle. In two minutes it had ceased to move, not having shewn any signs of excitement. It lay motionless, breathing at first deeply, afterwards more naturally. It was removed at the end of a quarter of an hour, and was found to be totally insensible. In five minutes it began to move, but rolled over in its first attempts to walk. Twenty minutes after its removal, it appeared to have recovered from the effects of the vapour.

Connected with the great volatility of this liquid is the increased quantity of it required to be present in the air to produce a given effect,—in accordance with the law which requires that the blood must be impregnated to a certain extent relatively to what it could imbibe. In one experiment I performed with this substance, one grain to each 100 cubic inches of air produced no appreciable effect whatever on a mouse confined for twenty minutes in it, although with that quantity of several less volatile bodies complete insensibility would have been induced.

In experiment 37 two grains to each 100 cubic inches of air produced the

* Vol. xli. p. 850.
† Edin. Med. and Surg. Jour., Oct. 1842.

second degree of narcotism; and in the following experiment four grains produced the fourth degree. The specific gravity of the vapour of bromide of ethyle is, I find, 3·78, the atom being represented by two volumes. Two grains will consequently occupy 1·706 cubic inches in the form of vapour. At the temperature of 100° the vapour of bromide of ethyle almost excludes the air, and occupies 92·8 per cent. of its place. So 1·706 ÷ 92·8 gives 0·0183, or nearly one fifty-fourth, as the relative saturation of the blood with this vapour for the second degree of narcotism; and there would be twice as much, or one twenty-seventh, for the fourth degree.

I have not ascertained by direct experiment how much bromide of ethyle serum will dissolve, but I find that water dissolves about one-sixtieth of its volume of it; and as the solubility of liquids of this kind is nearly the same in water as in serum, this may safely be taken as the standard;—when, if we consider the average quantity of serum in the human body to be 410 fluid ounces, as in a former part of these papers, and make the kind of calculation there made, we shall find that one fluid drachm and ten minims is the average quantity that there would be in the blood of a human subject in the second degree of narcotism; and two drachms and twenty minims in the fourth degree.

Dutch Liquid.

In recent works on chemistry this substance is called the hydrochlorate of chloride of acetyle. It is formed by the combination of equal volumes of olefiant gas and chlorine. It has a taste at once sweet and hot, and a pungent ethereal odour. It boils at 180°, and not at 148°, as Dr. Simpson states in some brief remarks on it in the Edinburgh Monthly Journal for April last, where he informs us that its vapour, when inhaled, causes so great irritation of the throat that few persons can persevere in inhaling it long enough to produce anæsthesia;. but that he had, however, " seen it inhaled perseveringly until this state, with all its usual phenomena, followed; and without excitement of the pulse or subsequent headache." My experiments with it have been confined to animals; and the two following will serve as a sample of them :—

Exp. 39.—One grain and a half of Dutch liquid was diffused through the air of a jar containing 400 cubic inches, and a mouse was introduced. After ten minutes had elapsed it began to stagger in its walk, and it continued to do so till it was removed at the end of half an hour. It was occasionally lying still, but always began to walk in an unsteady manner when the jar was moved. It was sensible to pinching on its removal, and in a quarter of an hour had recovered from its inebriation. It continued well.

Exp. 40.—A mouse was put into the same jar after three grains of Dutch liquid had been diffused in it. It began to stagger sooner than that employed in the last experiment ; and at the end of ten minutes had ceased to move, without having had any struggling or rigidity ; and it was not disturbed on the jar being moved. It lay breathing naturally till it was taken out at the end of half an hour, when it was found to be totally insensible to pinching. In ten minutes after its removal it began to move, but rolled over in its efforts to walk; when half an hour had elapsed it appeared to have recovered entirely from the narcotism, but was less lively than before ; and two or three hours afterwards it was observed to be suffering with difficulty of breathing, and it died in the course of the day. The lungs were congested and of a deep vermilion colour, probably the result of inflammation, occasioned by the irritating nature of the vapour. The right cavities of the heart were distended with dark-coloured coagulated blood. The same appearances were met with in another mouse that died in the same way after breathing this vapour.

In the first of these two experiments the second degree of narcotism was effected by three-eighths of a grain of vapour to each 100 cubic inches of air; and as the specific gravity of this vapour is 3·4484, three-eighths of a grain must occupy 0·35 of a cubic inch. I find that air, when saturated with vapour of Dutch liquid at 100°, contains 17·5 per cent., and therefore 0·35 ÷ 17·5 gives 0·02, or one-fiftieth, as the relative saturation of the blood in this degree. In the other experiment the fourth degree of narcotism was caused by twice as much vapour, or three-quarters of a grain to each 100 cubic inches, and, consequently, the blood would contain twice as much, or one twenty-fifth part of what it would hold in solution if saturated. I have ascertained that Dutch liquid requires about 100 parts of water for its solution, and taking its solubility in the serum to be the same, the blood would contain one part in 5000 in the second, and one part in 2500 in the fourth degree of narcotism, which in the human subject would be, on an average, 46 minims and 92 minims respectively.

General results of the experiments.

We have now seen the result of this experimental inquiry into the action of eight volatile substances, viz.: chloroform, ether, nitrate of oxide of ethyle, bisulphuret of carbon, benzin, bromoform, bromide of ethyle, and Dutch liquid. We find that the quantity of each substance in the blood, in corresponding degrees of narcotism, bears a certain proportion to what the blood would dissolve—a proportion that is almost exactly the same for all of them, with a slight exception in the case of benzin, which I believe is more apparent than real. The actual quantity of the different substances in the blood, however, differs widely; being influenced by their solubility. When the amount of saturation of the blood is the same, then it follows that the quantity of vapour required to produce the effect must increase with the solubility, and the effect produced by a given quantity must be in the inverse ratio of the solubility, as I announced some time ago.* This rule holds good with respect to all the substances of this kind that I have examined; including, in addition to those enumerated in this paper, bichloride of carbon, iodide of ethyle, acetate of oxide of ethyle, nitrate of oxide of methyle, acetate of oxide of methyle, pyroxilic spirit, acetone, and alcohol. The exact proportion in the blood, in the case of the three last mentioned, cannot be ascertained directly by experiments of the kind detailed above; for, being soluble to an unlimited extent, they continue to be absorbed as long as the experiment lasts: but from the large quantity of these substances that is required to produce insensibility, they confirm the rule stated above in a remarkable manner.

* MEDICAL GAZETTE, March 31.

This general law, of course, does not apply to all narcotics; not, for instance, to hydrocyanic acid, but only to those producing effects analogous to what are produced by ether, and having, I presume, a similar mode of action. I am not able at present to define them better than by calling them, that group of narcotics whose strength is inversely as their solubility in water (and consequently in the blood). In estimating their strength, when inhaled in the ordinary way, another element has to be taken into the account, viz., their volatility; for that influences the quantity that would be inhaled. By multiplying together the number of parts of water that each substance requires for its solution, and the number of minims of each substance that air will hold in solution at 60°, we get a set of figures expressive of the relative strength of each, when breathed in the ordinary way; and by another method of calculation the time might be expressed, in minutes and seconds, that it would take, on an average, to render persons, breathing in the usual way, insensible by each substance: but I shall here confine myself to enumerating the bodies I have examined in two columns; arranging them, in the first column, in the inverse order of their solubility, which is the direct order of their actual potency; and in the second column, in the order in which they stand after their volatility is taken into the account, which is the order of their potency when mixed with air till it is saturated at any constant temperature.

Bisulphuret of Carbon	Bisulphuret of Carbon
Bichloride of Carbon	Chloroform
Chloroform	Bichloride of Carbon
Bromoform	Bromoform
Benzin	Bromide of Ethyle
Dutch Liquid	Benzin
Iodide of Ethyle	Iodide of Ethyle
Bromide of Ethyle	Dutch Liquid
Nitrate of Oxide of Ethyle	Oxide of Ethyle (Ether)
Nitrate of Oxide of Methyle	Nitrate of Oxide of Ethyle
Oxide of Ethyle (Ether)	Nitrate of Oxide of Methyle
Acetate of Oxide of Ethyle	Acetate of Oxide of Ethyle
Acetate of Oxide of Methyle	Acetate of Oxide of Methyle
⎧ Acetone	Acetone
⎨ Pyroxilic Spirit	Pyroxilic Spirit
⎩ Alcohol	Alcohol

The general law, stated above, respecting the solubility of these liquids in the blood, applies also, with certain modifications, to a number of bodies which are gaseous at ordinary temperatures, and there are several important conclusions to be deduced from it. But before proceeding further in the attempt to give a general history of narcotic vapours and gases, and to determine what substances should be included in the list or otherwise, it will be well for me to describe, more particularly than I have done, the nature of the narcotism produced by the class of bodies we are considering, of which chloroform may very properly be taken as the type. I shall, therefore, next proceed to give the best description that I can of the effects of chloroform, having especially in view the practical importance of the agent; and shall make all the remarks that I am able to include in a brief space, on the administration of chloroform in surgical operations, medicine, and midwifery.

Description of the effects of Chloroform.

I may premise, that in applying the term narcotic to chloroform and other volatile substances, I employ it in the extended sense in which it is used by writers on materia medica and toxicology, who make it include all the substances which act on the nervous system; and I apply the term narcotism to designate all the effects of a narcotic, as I am entitled to do by strict etymology, and do not confine it, as the practice has generally been, to express a state of complete insensibility. I do not object to the term anæsthetic, but I use that of narcotic as being more comprehensive, and including the other properties of these vapours as well as that of annulling common sensibility.

To facilitate the description, I divide all the effects of chloroform short of the abolition of life, into five degrees. I use the term degree in preference to stage, as, in administering chloroform, the slighter degrees of narcotism occur in the latter stages of the process, during the recovery of the patient, as well as in the beginning.

The division into degrees is made according to symptoms, which, I believe, depend entirely on the state of the nervous centres, and not according to the amount of anæsthesia, which I shall give good reason for believing depends very much on local narcotism of the nerves.

In the first degree I include any effects of chloroform that exist while the patient possesses perfect consciousness of where he is, and what is occurring around him. As the sensations caused by inhaling a small quantity of chloroform have been experienced by nearly every medical man in his own person, I need not attempt to describe them. They differ somewhat with the individual, but may be designated as a kind of inebriation, which is usually agreeable when induced for curiosity, but is often otherwise, when the patient is about to undergo an operation: in such cases, however, this stage is very transitory. Although it is the property of narcotic vapours to suspend the functions of different parts of the nervous system in succession, yet they probably influence every part of that system from the first, but in different degrees.

I have found that my vision became impaired when inhaling chloroform, whilst I should have thought it as good as ever, had it not been that the seconds pointer disappeared from the watch on the table before me; and I could only discover it again by stooping to within a few inches within it. Common sensibility becomes also impaired, so that the pain of disease, which is generally due to a morbid increase of the common sensibility, is in many cases removed, or relieved, according to its intensity. And hence it is that patients are able to inhale chloroform and ether, without assistance, for the relief of neuralgia, dysmenorrhœa, and other painful affections; the latter, which acts less rapidly, being the best adapted for this kind of domestic use—chloroform being perhaps not perfectly safe. The sufferings attendant on parturition, when not unusually severe, may generally be prevented, as stated by Dr. Murphy,* without removing the patient's consciousness; but I have met with no instance in which the more severe kind of pain caused by the knife was prevented, whilst complete consciousness existed, except in a few cases, for a short time, as the patients were recovering from the effects of the va-

---

* Pamphlet on chloroform in the practice of midwifery.

pour, having just before been unconscious.

In the second degree of narcotism, there is no longer correct consciousness. The mental functions are impaired, but not altogether suspended. Generally, indeed, the patient neither speaks nor moves, but it is possible for him to do both; and this degree may be considered to be analogous to delirium, and to certain states of the patient in hysteria and concussion of the brain; and it corresponds with that condition of an inebriated person, who is not dead drunk, but in the state described by the law as drunk and incapable. It is so transitory, however, that the patient emerges to consciousness in a very few minutes at the farthest, if the chloroform is discontinued. This degree, any more than the others, cannot properly be compared to natural sleep, for the patient cannot be roused at any moment to his usual state of mind. Persons sometimes remember what occurs whilst they are in this state, but generally they do not. Any dreams that the patient has, occur whilst he is in this degree, or just going into, or emerging from it, as I have satisfied myself by comparing the expressions of patients with what they have related afterwards. There is generally a considerable amount of anæsthesia connected with this degree of narcotism, and I believe that it is scarcely ever necessary to proceed beyond it in obstetric practice, not even in artificial delivery, unless for the purpose of arresting powerful uterine action, in order to facilitate turning the fœtus. For, on the one hand, obstetric operations are less painful than those in which the knife is used, and, on the other, it is not so necessary that the patient should be perfectly motionless during their performance, as when the surgeon is cutting in the immediate vicinity of vital parts.* There is sometimes a considerable amount of mental excitement in this degree, rendering the patient rather unruly; but a further dose of the vapour removes this by inducing

the next degree of narcotism, and there is less difficulty from this source with chloroform than with ether, since its action is more rapid, and two or three inspirations often suffice to overcome the excitement. Very often, however, the patient is quiet, and to a certain extent tractable in this degree, and if sufficient anæsthesia can be obtained, there are certain advantages in avoiding to carry the narcotism beyond it for minor operations, especially tooth-drawing, as I shall explain when I enter on the uses and mode of applying chloroform, at the end of this sketch of its physiological effects. The patient is generally in this degree during the greater part of the time occupied in protracted operations; for, although, in most cases, it is necessary, as I have formerly stated, to induce a further amount of narcotism before the operation is commenced, it is not usually necessary to maintain it at a point beyond this.

The advent of the third degree of narcotism is marked by cessation of all voluntary motion. Usually the eyes become inclined upwards at the same time; and there is often a contracted state of the voluntary muscles, giving rise to more or less rigidity of the limbs. This contraction is greater and more frequent from chloroform than from ether, and, by affecting the muscles of the jaw, it sometimes causes a considerable obstacle to operations on the mouth. As there are no signs of ideas in this degree, I believe that there are none, and that the mental faculties are completely suspended: consequently the patient is perfectly secured against mental suffering from any thing that may be done. It does not follow, however, that an operation may always be commenced immediately the narcotism reaches this degree, for anæsthesia is not a necessary part of it; and unless the sensibility of the part to be operated on be suspended, or very much obscured, there may be involuntary movements sufficient to interfere with a delicate operation—not merely reflex movements, but also co-ordinate actions, such as animals may perform after the cerebral hemispheres are removed, the medulla oblongata being left. Under these circumstances an operation usually causes a contraction of the features expressive of pain, and sometimes moaning or cries, but

* Mr. Gream and Dr. Wm. Merriman, who have done me the honour of quoting from my essays on ether and chloroform, in their pamphlets, have applied to midwifery, what I meant to apply only to delicate and serious surgical operations, and have grounded objections on the supposed necessity of producing a deep state of narcotism.

D

not of an articulate kind. Whether or not these signs are to be considered proofs of pain, will depend on the definition given to the word; and if they do not interfere with the operator, or influence the recovery, they can be of no consequence, as there is no pain which has an existence for the patient. To obtain anæsthesia when it does not exist in this degree, and thus to prevent these symptoms if we desire, it is not necessary to carry the narcotism further, but only to wait at this point a few moments, giving a little chloroform occasionally to prevent recovery, and allow time for it to permeate the coats of the small vessels, and act more effectually on the nerves. The sensibility of the conjunctiva is a correct index of the general sensibility of the body; and until it is either removed or very much diminished, an operaion oft delicacy cannot be comfortably performed. Accordingly, in administering chloroform, as soon as the patient has inhaled sufficient to suspend voluntary motion, I raise the eyelid gently, touching its free border. If no winking is occasioned the operation may begin in any case, but if it is I wait a little time, till the eyelids either become quite passive or move less briskly. The state of the eye itself is observed, by this means, at the same time. It is usually turned up, and the pupil contracted, as Mr. Sibson has stated,* in the condition which I term the third degree of narcotism. The vessels of the conjunctiva, also, are sometimes injected, but more frequently they are not.

Dr. Hughes Bennet, in his able report on the properties of chloroform,† argues that the sensibility of the nerves is not suspended under its influence, because respiration, circulation, and uterine contractions continue, which could not be the case if the sensibility of the nerves connected with these functions were destroyed. This argument would have some weight if the nerves of common sensibility did not differ from those of the organic system, or those which arise from the respiratory tract of the medulla oblongata; but, as the case stands, it has none: and there is no more difficulty in conceiving a variable degree of susceptibility and of resistance to the effects of chloroform in different sets of nerves, than in different nervous centres. A careful observation of cases shows that the amount of local insensibility by no means keeps pace with the degree of sopor or coma, but is later in coming on and going off, and varies in amount in different patients; and as we know that chloroform, like other narcotics, produces some effect on parts to which it is locally applied, the conclusion seems irresistible, that it acts on the nerves as well as on the nervous centres. This view of the subject explains some circumstances which before seemed inexplicable; such as that of the patient recovering his consciousness, and telling the bystanders that he does not feel what is being done. For, whilst the vapour is escaping from the blood by way of the lungs, there is no difficulty in understanding how the brain may recover its influence sooner than the branches and peripheral expansion of the nerves; since, in the brain, not only is the circulation more rapid, but there is little, if any, lymph external to the vessels; whilst, in the body at large, the chloroform, having transuded through the coats of the capillaries into the extra-vascular liquor sanguinis, remains there for a little time, acting on the nervous fibrillæ, before it can pass again by endosmose into the vessels. It is in young subjects, in whom, connected with the more active process of nutrition, the quantity of lymph external to the vessels is greatest, that the general insensibility most frequently remains, whilst the cerebral hemispheres are resuming their functions.

In the fourth degree of narcotism there is relaxation of the voluntary muscles, together with general insensibility. I am better acquainted with this degree as induced by ether than by chloroform, for with the latter agent the third degree appears to encroach somewhat on this; chloroform seeming to differ from ether, and approaching somewhat in its effects to benzin and bisulphuret of carbon, which, we have seen, are not attended with muscular relaxation at any stage of their effects. Accordingly, I am inclined to prefer the use of ether, to assist the reduction of dislocations and strangulated herniæ.

---

* MED. GAZ., Feb. 18. I think that the turning up of the eyes is not so constant as Mr. Sibson believes, as I have been unable to observe it in some patients at any stage.

† Monthly Journal, Jan. 1848.

There is, however, often sufficient relaxation of the muscles to effect these objects even in the second degree of narcotism, especially if the effect have been kept up a little time. I was at one time inclined to believe that the functions of the spinal cord were more or less suspended in this degree, since reflex movements cannot be excited by any impressions made on the eyelids, or general surface of the body; but these reflex movements are absent in every degree of narcotism, when the common sensibility is abolished, and, therefore, the circumstance is best explained by attributing it to the narcotism of the nerves. Other functions of the spinal cord certainly remain; for the sphincters of the bladder and rectum continue contracted, and respiration goes on. The sensibility of the glottis continues, apparently unimpaired, in this degree of narcotism, but that of the pharynx is probably suspended; for, in operations on the mouth and nose, the blood sometimes finds its way into the stomach, without any visible act of swallowing. This takes place frequently, when the narcotism does not exceed the third degree. In these cases, it probably runs along the channel there is at each side of the epiglottis. The breathing is not unfrequently attended with some degree of stertor in the fourth degree; and the reason why one does not often meet with stertor in exhibiting chloroform, is, that one seldom carries the narcotism so far. There is a little stertor occasionally, even in the third degree of narcotism; and this symptom, and rigidity of the muscles, are met with altogether. There may be simple snoring in any degree of narcotism, and even in the natural sleep which often follows the state of insensibility; but it never comes on during the first minutes of the inhalation of chloroform, unless the narcotism reaches to the third or fourth degree. The iris is less sensible to light in this degree than under ordinary circumstances, and the pupil is about the usual size. I have never observed it widely dilated, or totally insensible to light.

I have not mentioned the pulse in the above outline of the action of chloroform on the human subject, as it is not indicative of the amount of narcotism. It is usually somewhat increased in force and frequency, as it is by a moderate amount of fermented liquor. This effect subsides with the effect of the vapour; but I have not remarked the pulse become slower after chloroform than it might be expected to be, in the same patient, in a state of perfect repose. 52 is the slowest pulse I have met with, and that was in a healthy man. This moderate acceleration is, I believe, the only direct effect of chloroform on the pulse. Indirectly, it may affect it in other ways. If, for instance, the breathing is interrupted by the pungency of the vapour, or from any other cause, the pulse becomes small and frequent, and when sickness is induced, it is diminished in force. If it is very frequent at the beginning of the inhalation, from mental perturbation, as is often the case, when the patient is about to undergo an operation, the frequency diminishes, as all anxiety departs with the loss of consciousness.

When animals are killed with chloroform, and not too abruptly, there is a stage between the fourth degree and the cessation of respiration in which the breathing is difficult, and sometimes slow and irregular. This I have named the fifth degree of narcotism. It is not every irregularity of breathing which is to be considered indicative of this degree,—for patients occasionally hold their breath for a short time, on account of the pungency of the vapour, and sometimes also, without any evident cause, in the second or third degree; but that need be no source of alarm. The fifth degree of narcotism, on the contrary, is the commencement of dying. I have only met with it in animals. It is sometimes accompanied with convulsive movements of the limbs—a result I never witnessed from ether.

Phenomena attending death from chloroform.

When the animal is made to breathe vapour of chloroform of such a strength that the respiration is stopped in the course of a few minutes, the heart continues to beat for a short time, and the circulation ceases only, as in asphyxia, for want of the respiration, without the heart having been brought under the influence of chloroform. The reason of this, as I explained, with respect to ether, on another occasion,* is not

---

* On the Inhalation of Ether, p. 81.

that the vapour is incapable of affecting the heart, but because a smaller quantity suffices to arrest the respiration, and the process of inhalation ceases, without the heart and blood-vessels being narcotised. The two following experiments illustrate and prove these points :—

Exp. 41.—A nearly full-grown rabbit was placed in a jar containing 1600 cubic inches, with 64 grs. of chloroform, being four grains to each 100 cubic inches. At first it tried to get out, afterwards it struggled involuntarily, and then sank slowly down, and lay, when four minutes had elapsed, in a flaccid condition, breathing naturally. It did not stir afterwards, except from a slight convulsive twitch of its paw once or twice. In three or four minutes more, the breathing became slower, and ten minutes after it was put in, it breathed its last. It was immediately taken out, and the stethoscope applied to the chest. The heart was heard to beat for between two and three minutes, at first nearly as rapidly as before the experiment, but more slowly and less audibly towards the end. The chest was opened a few minutes afterwards, and feeble rhythmic contractions of both auricles and ventricles were observed, not strong enough to expel the blood with which the heart was filled, but not to distension. These contractions continued unabated during the half hour the inspection continued. The lungs were perfectly healthy, and not congested. Next morning the body was rigid, and the blood in the heart and adjoining vessels coagulated. The sinuses in the cranium were filled with blood, and the vessels on the surface of the brain were somewhat injected, but not those in its substance.

Exp. 42.—Four and a half grains of chloroform were introduced into a jar containing 600 cubic inches, being three-quarters of a grain to each 100 cubic inches, and, the vapour having been equally diffused, two frogs were put in. They tried to climb up the side of the jar, as if wishing to make their escape, and one or the other occasionally ceased to breathe for a minute or two, probably from disliking the vapour, but commenced to breathe again. In about five minutes the efforts to escape ceased, and they only moved to adjust their equilibrium when the jar was disturbed. They were now breathing regularly, and continued to do so till about ten minutes after their introduction, when all voluntary power ceased, and the breathing began to be performed only at intervals. They were allowed to remain till half an hour had elapsed, during the last ten minutes of which time no respiratory movement was observed in either of them. On taking them out, and laying them on their backs, the pulsations of the heart were observed on each side of the sternum. These pulsations were the more distinct from the lungs being apparently empty. Now an experiment with chloroform on the frog does not necessarily cease with its pulmonary respiration, for it is capable of both absorbing and giving off vapour by the skin. Accordingly I continued the experiment on these frogs, placing one of them back again, in the course of two or three minutes, in the same jar, with three grains of chloroform, and the other in a jar of 400 cubic inches capacity, with five grains. They were laid on their backs, and the heart of the former one, in air containing half a grain of chloroform to each 100 cubic inches, continued to beat distinctly and regularly, 45 times in the minute, for four hours that it remained in the jar, and it was not observed to breathe during the whole time, although it was watched almost constantly. The respiration commenced again within half an hour after its removal. In about an hour it recovered its power of voluntary motion, and it was not injured by the long narcotism.

The pulsations of the heart of the other frog, in air containing a grain and a quarter of chloroform to each 100 cubic inches of air, became slower and more feeble, and in a quarter of an hour could not be observed. The frog was left in the jar a quarter of an hour longer, and removed when it had been in half an hour. The under part of the thorax was immediately opened sufficiently to expose the heart. It was moderately full of blood, but not contracting at all, and it did not evince the least irritability on being pricked, either now or after exposure to the air for some time. It is evident that the heart of this last frog became paralysed by the absorption into the blood of more vaponr, in addition to the quantity that was sufficient to arrest the respiration. The temperature of the room during this experiment was 65°.

The effect of chloroform on the heart of the frog is further shewn by the next experiment.

Exp. 43.—A frog was placed in the jar containing 600 cubic inches, with six grains of chloroform. In twenty minutes the respiration had ceased, but the heart continued to . pulsate strongly. At the end of three-quarters of an hour the pulsations were more feeble, and had diminished from 40 to 30 in the minute. An hour and five minutes from the commencement of the experiment, no movement of the heart could be observed. The frog was taken out of the vapour, and a portion of the sternum and integuments removed, so as partly to expose the heart, when it was found to be still contracting, with a very feeble undulatory motion. This motion increased in force, and, in a quarter of an hour after its removal, the heart was pulsating regularly and strongly, the ventricle apparently emptying itself perfectly. When the frog had been out twenty minutes, it was placed again in the same jar, with the same quantity of chloroform. In about ten minutes the heart's action began to fail again, and in about twenty minutes the slightest movement could no longer be perceived in it. The frog was immediately taken out, and the ventricle of the heart was pricked with a needle. In a few seconds a slight quivering was observed,—whether the result of the prick is not certain, and the action of the heart became gradually re-established as before. It was arrested a third time by exposure to the vapour; and although, in its third removal, the anterior extremities of the frog had become rigid, the heart resumed its action partially, and continued to contract feebly for three or four hours after the rigidity of death had invaded the body and limbs of the animal.* The temperature of the room was 62° during this experiment.

We learned from some of the experiments detailed in the early part of this paper, that the presence in the blood

* The setting in of rigidity in the frog is accompanied by a partial change of posture, and the contraction is sometimes strong enough to move the whole body.

of one twenty-second part as much chloroform as it would dissolve, had the effect of arresting the respiration. From the last experiment we can determine how much it takes to stop the action of the heart. One grain of chloroform, as was stated before, produces 0·767 of a cubic inch of vapour; and at 62°— the temperature during this experiment—air, when saturated, contains 13·8 cubic inches. Therefore 0·767÷13·8 gives 0·0555, or one-eighteenth of what the blood would dissolve as the quantity which has the effect of arresting the heart's action.

———

Phenomena attending death from Chloroform. — Post-mortem appearances. —The fatal cases of inhalation of Chloroform.

In my last communication it was shewn, that when an animal of warm blood is made to breathe the vapour of chloroform, well diluted with air, until death ensues, the heart continues to pulsate for some time after the respiration has ceased, the circulation being arrested, secondarily, by the failure of the breathing. It was also shewn, by some experiments on frogs, that chloroform has the effect of directly paralyzing the heart, when it is absorbed in a somewhat larger quantity than is required to stop the respiratory movements. It is possible, indeed, to narcotise the heart of warm-blooded animals by chloroform. When the vapour is exhibited to them in a concentrated form, the breathing and circulation appear to cease nearly together; probably, because the quantity of vapour in the lungs, at the time the breathing stops, is sufficient, when absorbed, and added to that already in the blood, to narcotise the heart. The two following experiments confirm this view.

Exp. 44.—120 grains of chloroform were put into a jar of the capacity of 600 cubic inches, which was kept accurately covered with a piece of plate-glass, and moved about to diffuse the chloroform over its sides. In a few minutes the chloroform was all converted into vapour. The temperature of the jar was 65°, the air in it was consequently nearly saturated with vapour, and contained 20 grains in each 100 cubic inches. A young rabbit was put into the jar. It was very quickly affected, and ceased to breathe in less than a minute. It was taken out immediately the respiration ceased, and the ear was applied to its chest, but no motion of the heart was audible. The thorax was opened as quickly as possible, and when the heart was first observed it was quite motionless; but it had not been exposed to the air for a minute, before it began to contract, the auricles beginning to move first, and shortly afterwards the ventricles,—and in three or four minutes it was contracting vigorously. This recommencement of the heart's action no doubt resulted from the evaporation of the chloroform from its surface, and the consequent liberation of the nerves there situated from the influence of the vapour. Soon after the chest had been opened, a drop of chloroform was allowed to fall on the heart, and its motion instantly ceased, but gradually commenced again in the course of a few minutes, and it continued to contract feebly for some time. The lungs, which collapsed as soon as the chest was opened, were, when first observed, of a vermilion tint. This colour of the lungs is an additional proof that the circulation had not continued after the respiration ceased. There was active vermicular motion of the intestines of the rabbit when they were exposed to the air, soon after death, and a drop of chloroform being put on the ileum at once stopped the contractions at the place of contact, whilst they continued as before in the rest of the intestine. The next morning the body of the rabbit was rigid, and the blood in the heart was coagulated. The right cavities were nearly full, and the left contained a small quantity of blood. The brain was quite healthy, its vessels not being congested.

EXP. 45.—Two fluid drachms of chloroform were put into the same jar, which was placed near the fire, and moved about till the liquid was all converted into vapour, when the air within was of the temperature of 75°, saturated with chloroform, and containing about 29 grains in each 100 cubic inches. A young rabbit was put in. It first attempted to escape, then gave a little cry, and sank down on its side, and was dead three quarters of a minute after its introduction. It was immediately removed, and the ear applied to its chest, but no sound could be heard. The thorax was opened directly, and the heart observed to be perfectly motionless; but it commenced to contract after its exposure, as in the former experiment, and in a few minutes was contracting vigorously. The rabbit was placed back again in the jar, in which the vapour was still retained, except a little that escaped during the momentary removal of the cover, and the heart became quickly affected from the absorption of the vapour by its moist surface. Its contractions became more and more feeble, and at the end of four minutes had entirely ceased, and could not be excited by pricking; yet they commenced again spontaneously about ten minutes after the removal of the rabbit from the jar, but were not so strong as before. The lungs of this rabbit were of a vermilion colour when the chest was opened, and the appearances on examination of the body next day were precisely the same as in the former experiment.

It has appeared to me that the respiration and circulation cease nearly together in those instances, also, in which an animal is slowly killed by the inhalation of vapour of chloroform of moderate strength. One experiment will suffice to relate in illustration of this.

EXP. 46.—A cat, which it was requisite to destroy, was placed in a jar holding 800 cubic inches, and a fluid drachm and a half of chloroform was put in, and the jar covered. The cat made efforts to escape for the first minute; it then became insensible, and was affected with spasmodic movements for about half a minute, after which it was quite motionless, and relaxed, and the breathing ceased about two minutes after the commencement of the experiment. It was taken out, and the stethoscope applied to the chest, and the sounds of the heart's action were distinctly heard. At this moment the breathing began again, and the cat was put back into the jar, from which, however, the greater part of the vapour had escaped. It remained insensible, and the breathing after a time became very feeble, except at intervals, when it was laborious. In little more than half an hour the animal died. It was taken out as soon as the respiration ceased, but no movement of the heart could be heard. Next day the body was very rigid, the right cavities of the heart and the two cavæ were full, but not greatly distended; the left cavities of the heart were nearly empty. All the blood was dark coloured and fluid. The lungs were collapsed and of a bright red colour. They were not congested.

Post-mortem appearances.

As might be expected from these investigations concerning the mode in which chloroform causes death, the post-mortem appearances resulting from it are neither constant nor striking. I have preserved brief notes of the examination of 14 animals killed by chloroform—3 cats, 3 rabbits, 2 guinea pigs, 4 small birds (chaffinches and larks), and 2 mice. In every instance the right cavities of the heart were more or less filled with blood, and in five cases out of the fourteen they were much distended. The left cavities of the heart contained a little blood in every instance in which their state is mentioned. The blood was fluid in one instance—that of the cat, related above. In the other instances it was coagulated—generally firmly, but in three or four cases only loosely. The lungs were quite free from congestion in ten of the animals, in the other four they were congested in patches. The head was examined in only eight instances, and in these the substance of the brain was free from congestion, and the sinuses were not particularly distended, except in two.

The fatal cases of inhalation of chloroform.

After seeing how rapidly the vapour of chloroform kills animals when it pervades to a certain extent the air they breathe, and when we recollect that it came all at once to be generally administered without any previous teaching on the subject in the schools, it ought not to surprise us, however much we are called on to deplore the circumstance, that a few cases have occurred, in different parts of the world, in which the exhibition of chloroform has been attended with fatal results; especially when we consider that the vapour has usually been so administered that its strength could not be controlled. Reflecting, indeed, on the mildness and uniformity of the action of the vapour on animals, when more diluted, as shown in some of the experiments related in the first part of these papers, we ought to feel confident that it is capable of being used with perfect safety, certainty, and precision; and this view of the subject agrees with my experience, which has extended now over a great number of cases.

I offered some remarks at the time respecting the fatal case that occurred near Newcastle.* The next case recorded is one at Cincinnati, U. S. in February last.† The remarks I made on the Newcastle case apply in a great measure to this. Although the chloroform was not administered on a handkerchief, the vapour seems to have been inhaled in too concentrated a form, as its effects were produced very rapidly. The patient inhaled from a glass globe, containing a sponge of considerable size saturated with chloroform. "Breathing at first slow; inhaled 12 or 15 times, occupying from a minute to 75 seconds," and some stumps of teeth were then immediately removed. Now, it takes three or four moderately deep inspirations, and as many expirations, to replace all the air contained at one time in the lungs. Consequently, the patient was made sufficiently insensible for the operation by the effect of about 8 to 12 inspirations, whilst the chloroform of 3 or 4 inspirations more was in the lungs, waiting to be absorbed and increase the effect. I am aware that part of this would be expired again unabsorbed as the patient continued to breathe, but that is equally true of what was inhaled at the previous inspirations; so the fact remains, that the patient must have had from one-third to one-half more chloroform than was necessary to produce what was deemed sufficient insensibility. And according to what I have observed, insensibility to pain cannot be obtained in a very rapid manner without considerable narcotism of the nervous centres—the third or fourth degree: therefore, that the patient should be in a dying state a few moments after the inhalation was discontinued, was only what might have been expected. The female friends of the patient considered that she died about two minutes after the commencement of the inhalation; and although the dentists who administered the chloroform thought that the patient lived a few minutes longer, yet, even according to their account, she was during this time in a dying condition. According to

---

* MED. GAZ. vol xli. p. 277.
† Ibid. vol. xlii. p. 79.

Mrs. Pearson's account, which is clear and precise, the pulse became feeble and then stopped, and the breathing ceased about the same time. This agrees with what is stated above respecting the phenomena of death when rapidly caused by chloroform, and with what was observed in the rabbits in experiments 44 and 45.

On inspecting the body, the brain was found to be in a normal state, but the vessels and sinuses of the dura mater contained a larger quantity of blood than usual, which was liquid, and mixed with some bubbles of air. The lungs were considerably, but not intensely, congested. The heart was flaccid, and all its cavaties entirely empty. It had been emptied, undoubtedly, after death. Artificial respiration was resorted to, and Mr. Sibson has remarked * that he has often known the heart to be emptied after death by artificial inflation of the lungs. Or if the head was first opened, as appears by the order in which the inspection is reported, part of the two or three ounces of fluid blood which flowed from the sinuses of the dura mater might have come from the right side of the heart, as I have seen the blood flow from the chest and out by the lateral sinuses in an inspection in which it was liquid. The blood in the case under consideration was as fluid as water in every part of the body, and the globules were thought to be altered in microscopic appearance. The causes which prevent the coagulation of the blood after death are not yet well understood, and although it is not correct, as was once supposed, that fluidity of the blood is a constant rule in certain kinds of sudden death, yet there are sufficient cases recorded where it was so, to show that it is not uncommon in the human subject when death takes place suddenly. The observations on animals, recorded above, as well as numerous others, show that it is not a characteristic property of chloroform to prevent the coagulation of the blood; and I think that the artificial respiration would assist, in more ways than one, to prevent its coagulation in this case, and one presently to be mentioned.

The next case that we have to notice occurred at Hyderabad.† The subject

of it was a young woman, who required to have the distal phalanx of one of her fingers amputated. The surgeon who operated says, " I administered a drachm of chloroform in the usual way —namely, by sprinkling it on a pocket handkerchief, and causing her to inhale the vapour. She coughed a little, and then gave a few convulsive movements." When these subsided, the operation was performed, and endeavours were made to recover the patient, but in vain. Scarcely a drop of blood escaped during the operation, and the surgeon remarks, " I am inclined to think that death was almost instantaneous; for, after the convulsive movements above described, she never moved, or exhibited the smallest sign of life." There was no inspection of the body.

The case which occurred at Boulogne,* is so like the above, that we may consider the two together. The patient was a female, about 30 years of age, and took chloroform for the opening of an abscess. M. Gorré, the operator, says, " I placed over the nostrils of the patient, a handkerchief moistened with from fifteen to twenty drops at the most of chloroform. Scarcely had she taken several inspirations, when she put her hand on the handkerchief to withdraw it, and cried with a plaintive voice, " I choak !" Immediately the face became pale; [a symptom recorded also of the Newcastle case; and the one at Cincinnati] the countenance changed; the breathing embarrassed; and she foamed at the mouth. At the same instant, (and that certainly less than a minute after the beginning of the inhalation), the handkerchief moistened with chloroform was withdrawn." The operation was performed, and then efforts were made to restore the patient, but she was dead; and M. Gorré remarks that the death was without doubt complete at the moment when he made the incision.

From experiments related in former parts of these papers, the conclusion was arrived at, that to produce a degree of narcotism that would arrest the respiration, the blood must contain about one twenty-second part as much chloroform as it would dissolve; and that to narcotise the heart so as to stop its contractility, the blood must contain

---

* MED. GAZ. vol. xlii. p. 216.
† Ibid. p. 84.

* See MED. GAZ. vol. xlii. p. 76 and 211.

about one-eighteenth part as much as it would dissolve. By a calculation similar to that made before,* I find that half a fluid drachm is the quantity that there should be in the whole of the blood of a person of average size, to stop the respiration, and 37 minims to arrest the heart's action. In the case which occurred in India, a drachm of chloroform was placed on the handkerchief. We cannot easily suppose that more than half of this entered the patient's lungs, since the expired air carries away a portion as it passes over the handkerchief. And since, as was estimated before, only about half of what enters the lungs becomes absorbed, the remainder being expired again, there could only be about fifteen minims in the blood. This quantity, supposing the young Hindoo female was but half the average size of the adult, and this is not improbable, would only be just sufficient to cause death by arresting the respiration, without immediately stopping the heart's action, providing the chloroform were equally diffused through the whole of the blood. There is every reason, however, from the symptoms, to believe that the action of the heart was suddenly arrested; and the quantity used in the case at Boulogne would not have sufficed to cause death in any way, if it had been equally mixed with the blood. But it was not equally diffused through the circulation in either case,—there was not time for it to be so. Mr. Sibson, in treating the subject of death from chloroform,† makes some remarks in which I entirely agree. He says, " the poison penetrates to the heart from the lungs in a single pulsation, and at the beginning of the next systole the blood is sent through the coronary artery to the whole muscular tissue of the heart. The blood passing into the coronary artery is less diluted—is more strongly impregnated with chloroform—than is the blood in any other part of the system, except the lungs." By experiments 42 to 45 on frogs and rabbits, it has been shewn that chloroform will act locally on the heart; consequently, if the blood passing from the lungs to the left side of the heart should happen to contain one-eighteenth part as

much vapour as it would dissolve, the patient might be suddenly killed before the nervous system in general were brought under the influence of the narcotic. A small quantity of chloroform might suffice to produce this result, if the vapour were mixed with only a limited portion of air.

The difficulty of inhaling the vapour in a concentrated form, on account of its pungency, and the further dilution of it when inhaled with the air already in the lungs, no doubt would usually prevent this kind of accident, and are in fact the reasons why it has not more often occurred. Still I believe that the patient is not safe unless the vapour is systematically mixed with so much air that no great quantity of it can be in the lungs at one time. I am of opinion that ether is incapable of causing this kind of accident; for the blood may imbibe with safety so considerable a volume of its vapour, that the quantity which the lungs can contain at once, adds but little to the effect. And I consider that a patient could only lose his life by ether, from its careless continuance for several inspirations after well-marked symptoms of danger had set in.

M. Gorré says that he poured on the handkerchief not more than fifteen to twenty drops. The drops of chloroform are very small. When dropped from an ordinary phial, nine of them are equal to about two minims, and twenty drops would be less than five minims—a very small quantity. But, as the chloroform was poured, he probably means as much as would be equal to fifteen or twenty drops of water—in fact, about as many minims; and, indeed, as it was not measured, we have no means of being certain that there was not more—say, half a fluid-drachm. However, fifteen minims might be amply sufficient to cause death in the way indicated above, even if but half of it entered the lungs; and the sudden paleness, and almost instantaneous death, clearly indicate that the circulation must have ceased suddenly.

The post-mortem appearances in the case at Boulogne were very nearly the same as in the case which occurred at Cincinnati, previously alluded to. Artificial respiration had been resorted to, and carried to the extent of permanently dilating the pulmonary vesicles.

* MED. GAZ. vol. xli. p. 894.
† Ibid. vol. xlii. p. 109.

E

Air was met with in the sinuses of the dura mater in the American case, and in this case a good deal of air was mixed with the blood in the veins of almost all parts of the body. There can be but little doubt that this was a result of the artificial respiration, although one cannot tell precisely in what way the result was produced. The peculiar state of the blood, which was very fluid and dark-coloured, as in the American case, must have depended rather on the suddenness of the death, and the artificial respiration, than on any immediate action of the small quantity of chloroform—a quantity much less than is usually inhaled in a surgical operation.

A patient died whilst taking chloroform during an amputation at the hipjoint, at the Hôpital Beaujon, in Paris. But the death in this instance was probably not entirely due to the chloroform; for although the patient apparently got an overdose of the vapour when it was repeated during the operation, yet, as the pulse was occasionally appreciable for three-quarters of an hour afterwards, he would most likely have recovered, had it not been for the lesion occasioned by the operation, which it seems was never finished. So the four cases previously alluded to, and which happened at Newcastle, Cincinnati, Hyderabad, and Boulogne respectively, comprise the whole of the instances in which it appears to me that death has clearly and undoubtedly resulted from the inhalation of chloroform. There was a death at Aberdeen, but not from the professional administration of the agent. There is another case, however, in which the death is generally attributed to the chloroform; and occurring, as it did, in the practice of Mr. Robinson, who has had great experience, and deservedly earned a high reputation, connected with the administration of ether and chloroform, it has made a great impression both on medical men and the public. My reasons for doubting that death was caused by chloroform in this instance are these:—Mr. Robinson's servant states, in her evidence, that the inhaler was not applied to the patient's face, but held at a little distance from it; and, with the kind of inhaler Mr. Robinson uses, it is impossible that the air the patient breathed could become strongly charged with vapour in this way; for it would pass into the mouth and nostrils by the side of the face-piece, and very little of it would pass over or through the sponge. Again, the patient was remarking that the vapour was not strong enough, just when the inhaler was removed, and the moment before he suddenly expired.* I consider that he would have made no such remark if there had been a quantity of vapour in his lungs capable of suddenly paralysing the heart. This condition of the patient is totally unlike the coughing and convulsions in the case in India, or the exclamation "I choke," in that at Boulogne. I am not inclined, however, to attribute the sudden death at that moment to a mere coincidence, as it might be occasioned by mental emotion. Fainting is not altogether peculiar to the female sex; and, supposing syncope to occur in a patient who has fatty degeneration of the substance of the heart, and an enlarged liver greatly encroaching on the space of the thorax, one can easily understand why he should not recover. In some of the reports it was stated that the patient did not appear alarmed, for he was laughing and talking the moment before he died; but I do not know why a patient should laugh in a dentist's operating chair, unless to disguise or try to banish his apprehension. He had been led by his medical attendant in the country to believe that the chloroform would be attended with danger in his case; and again, just the moment before he died, Mr. Robinson was asking him to have his teeth taken out without proceeding further with the vapour. The post-mortem appearances are quite consistent with this cause of death; and, according to this view of the subject, the disease of the internal organs assists to explain the fatal occurrence; but I do not see how it can assist in explaining it, if it be attributed to chloroform, although I am aware that it is usually thought to do so.

If the heart were so thinned that it were in danger of being ruptured by the least distension, or if some of its orifices were so contracted that it

---

* I do not understand why Mr. Robinson was proceeding to add more chloroform, having previously put a drachm and a half on the sponge, as applying the inhaler closer to the face would have made the vapour stronger.

could not maintain the circulation under increased exertion or excitement, I could understand how the inhalation might be attended with danger, if excitement and struggling were produced by it, as sometimes happens. And on these grounds I always looked on extensive disease of the heart as a contra-indication, to a certain extent, of inhalation, and have expressed opinions to that effect; but I cannot conceive how a moderate and gradual inhalation of chloroform should cause any person's heart, however diseased, suddenly to cease beating. There are neither facts nor analogies in support of such an occurrence. Mr. Thomas Wakley, having met with great congestion of the heart and lungs in certain of the animals that he killed with chloroform, and mistaking, in my opinion, the consequence of the mode of dying for the cause of death, had expressed an opinion that this agent would be particularly dangerous in diseases of the heart and lungs; but this case, the only one of those where death was attributed to chloroform, in which any previous disease of these organs was found, cannot be considered to support an opinion founded on these grounds; for here there was no congestion of the heart, and but very little of the lungs. I am happy to find views similar to my own, respecting chloroform in disease of the heart, entertained by one whose opinion, both on account of the attention he has paid to this subject, and his great merit as a physiologist, is entitled to so much respect as that of Mr. Sibson. He says* that "persons the subject of heart disease, when the dread of a severe operation is great, may sometimes be peculiarly benefited by the careful and short production of anæsthesia during the cutting part of an operation."

On the administration of chloroform—Objections to giving it on a handkerchief— Description of an apparatus.

THE conclusion generally arrived at by those who have commented on the fatal cases of inhalation of chloroform, is one in which I do not agree. It has usually been concluded that there

* Loc. cit.

is danger necessarily attending the use of chloroform, and that it should therefore be confined to serious operations. Now a great part of the advantage attending the use of an anæsthetic consists in its preventing the patient's dread of the operation; but if the immunity from pain could only be obtained by incurring a danger of sudden loss of life, there would be a new source of fear. Many patients, again, have been readily induced to submit to a necessary operation, through the prospect of undergoing it without pain, who, otherwise, would have withheld their consent either altogether or till the prospect of a successful issue were much diminished. In this way, there is no doubt, many lives have been saved. But if the patient had to choose between pain and a risk, however small, of sudden death, this ready and early consent could not be expected. It is therefore necessary, for the sake of patients undergoing capital operations, to inquire whether there is any means of preventing the pain, which is free from danger, and to employ that means in preference to another. And if the skilful and careful administration of chloroform were really attended with danger, I would recommend that it should not be resorted to in any case; for we have in ether a medicine capable of affording all the benefits that can be derived from chloroform, and which never caused accidents of the kind we are considering, although it was the first used,—when the knowledge, consequently, of producing insensibility was less.*

There is, however, no reason to doubt that chloroform is, when administered with care and a sufficient knowledge of its properties, unattended with danger,—or, at all events, with a degree of danger so small that it cannot

* I am aware that ether was thought by some to have caused death in two or three instances in which the patients did not recover from the operation, but died two or three days afterwards; and in one of these instances a coroner's jury returned a verdict to that effect; but I believe the only instance on record in which the inhalation of ether was fatal, was one that occurred in France (see Gaz. Médicale, 4 Mars, and MED. GAZ. p. 432, last vol.), and in that case the inhalation was continued without intermission for ten minutes, although alarming symptoms were present nearly all the time; and it is probable that the result was owing as much to some defect in the inhaler, which limited the supply of air, as to the effect of ether.

be estimated;—not greater, for instance, than attends the minor operations of surgery, or the taking of ordinary doses of medicine. When the vapour of chloroform is well diluted with air, it is as safe as ether; and, as it possesses some minor advantages over it,—such as being less pungent, and therefore more easily inhaled,—not leaving its odour in the breath for some time afterwards,—being more portable, on account of the smaller quantity required, and producing excitement less frequently in the early stages of its effects,—its use, by all medical men who are perfectly conversant with its effects and mode of administration, is quite allowable in every case in which there is much pain to be prevented.

But, without proper precautions, the inhalation of chloroform is undoubtedly attended with danger, on account of the rapidity of its action when not sufficiently diluted with air, and, also, on account of its effects accumulating for about twenty seconds after it is discontinued, which accumulation would be most formidable, if the air taken into the lungs just before, were highly charged with vapour. The exhibition of ether is not attended with this kind of danger, even if but little precaution is exercised, and the symptoms caused by both vapours being the same, I entirely agree in the recommendation of M. Valleix, physician to the Hôtel Dieu, that medical men who have not practised anæsthesia should first study it from the action of ether.* This advice will, perhaps, not generally be followed; but if practitioners are inclined to run any risk in administering chloroform before they are well prepared, they must recollect that they are not doing it for the sake of preventing the severe pain and shock of the operation, but only to avoid the stronger odour, more pungent flavour, and other little inconveniences of ether.

It is quite obvious, that by merely placing the chloroform on a handkerchief or sponge, and getting the patient to breathe through it, we can have no control over the quantity of vapour in the air breathed. If the handkerchief be not applied close to the face, enough vapour will, most likely, not be taken to cause insensibility; and, if applied closely, the air breathed will probably be almost saturated, and that at a rather high temperature. In three out of the four fatal cases we have considered, the chloroform was administered on a handkerchief; and in the fourth case —that in America—no attention was paid to the proportions of vapour and air: the only endeavour appeared to be to make the patient insensible as quickly as possible. The handkerchief is advocated by some practitioners, on account of its supposed simplicity; but whenever I have had occasion to give chloroform in this way, I have felt it to be a very complicated process, on account of the difficulty of getting even an approximative knowledge of what I was doing, by the best calculation I could make.

Before administering chloroform, the surgeon should have as clear and distinct an idea of its vapour as of the blade of his knife; and as this will be read by students as well as practitioners, I shall be excused for introducing a brief explanation of the nature of a vapour. In a popular sense, this term is sometimes applied to the minute globules of liquid suspended in air, which result from the condensation of a vapour that has been mixed with it, as in what is called the steam or vapour from the spout of a tea-kettle. But chloroform cannot be taken in this form; if it were attempted, spasm of the glottis would ensue. A vapour is a dry aeriform condition of a substance differing from a gas only in the circumstances of temperature and pressure under which it takes the liquid form. The vapour of chloroform has no separate existence under natural circumstances of pressure and temperature, or in any form of inhaler. No patient ever took any of it in this way, or ever will, and this is equally true of ether.* Chloroform requires a

---

* See MED. GAZ. p. 305, present vol.

* Many practitioners, judging from their writings, seem to have very incorrect notions concerning these vapours. For instance, M. Roux, the eminent French surgeon, in objecting to the use of the handkerchief in the Academy of Sciences, says—" In this manner the patient inspires the chloroform vapour without air. (See MED. GAZ. present vol. p. 214). Soon after the inhalation of ether was introduced, two veterinary surgeons in London endeavoured to try its effects on a horse in a pure state, and prevented the ingress of air. As they did not make the ether boil, the animal could get no vapour, except what com-

temperature of 140° Fah., under the ordinary pressure of the atmosphere, to make it boil, and enable it to exist in the state of undiluted vapour; but mixed with air, it may have the form of vapour at inferior temperatures : the quantity that may exist in the air varying with the temperature directly as the elastic force of the vapour. The chloroform, in fact, that a patient breathes, is dissolved in the air, just as water is always dissolved in it, even in the driest weather, and the patient breathes his air with two vapours instead of one—the new vapour being, to be sure, in much the largest quantity. As a proof that these physical considerations are worthy our notice, I may state, that if chloroform had boiled at 180° instead of 140°, its solubility and other properties remaining the same, the four fatal cases we had occasion to discuss would not have occurred.

The following table shews the result of experiments I made to determine the quantity of vapour of chloroform that 100 cubic inches of air will take up at various temperatures :—

Temperature.	Cubic inches.
50°	9
55	11
60	14
65	19
70	24
75	29
80	36
85	44
90	55

The most perfect way of giving a vapour to animals is that adopted in the experiments I have related, the breathing not being interfered with, and the strength of the vapour being accurately known. This method is not applicable to patients, but our endeavour should be to approach to it as nearly as we conveniently can. The apparatus I employ is delineated in the subjoined engraving.* (See next page).

bined with the little air that might get in through the leakage of the inhaler. The horse in fact was burked. The efforts at respiration were prodigious,—it shortly died,—and the heart and diaphragm were found to be ruptured. (See Lancet, April 10, 1847). This experiment has been recently quoted in a pamphlet opposed to chloroform in midwifery, as a proof of the injurious effects of ether.

* It is made according to my directions, by Mr. Matthews, 10, Portugal Street, Lincoln's Inn Fields,

a. Outer case containing water bath, screwed on—*b.* Cylindrical vessel into which the chloroform is put; it is lined with a coil or two of bibulous paper up to the point *c d.* A cylindrical frame which screws into *b*—it has apertures at the top for the admission of air, and its lower two-thirds are covered with a coil or two of bibulous paper, which touches the bottom of the vessel *b*, except where the notches *e* are cut in it. *f.* Elastic tube. *g.* Expiratory valve of face piece; the dotted lines indicate the position of this valve when turned aside for the admission of air not charged with vapour. *h.* Inside view of face-piece, pinched together at the top to adapt it to a smaller face. *i.* Inspiratory valve.

When the patient inspires, the air enters by the numerous and large apertures in the top of the inhaler, passes between the two cylinders of bibulous paper, wet with chloroform, through the notches in the bottom of the inner one, then up the centre of the apparatus, still in contact with the paper, and through the short tube, which is three-quarters of an inch wide in the inside. The air thus gets charged with vapour, whilst it meets with no obstruction whatever till it arrives at the inspiratory valve of vulcanized India-rubber, which weighs but a few grains, and rises at the beginning of the slightest possible inspiratory movement. The cylinder of thin brass in which the chloroform is placed is inclosed in a larger one containing water, which, by supplying the caloric that is removed in the vaporization of the medicine, prevents the temperature from being lowered. It also prevents it from being raised by the warmth of the hand, and thus keeps the process steady. If the temperature of the water be 60°, each 100 cubic inches of air passing through the apparatus might, according to the table above, take up 14 cubic inches, and become expanded to 114 cubic inches, when it would contain a little more than twelve per cent. by measure. This is supposing it became quite saturated, which, however, it does not, and ten per cent. of vapour, or eight minims of chloroform, is probably as much as the air contains. It is not desirable, however, to give it to the patient even of this strength, and the

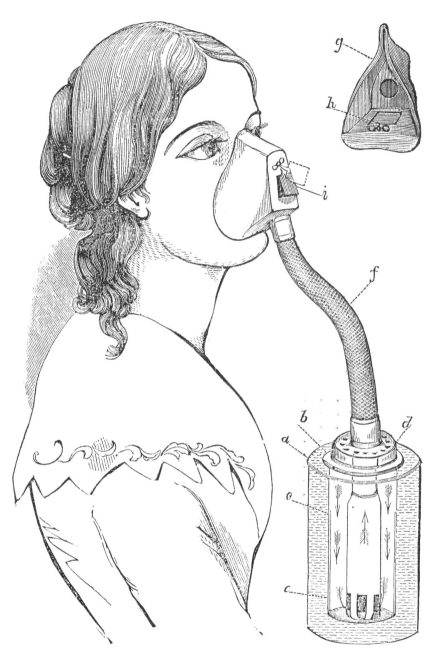

expiratory valve of the face-piece * is made to move to one side, so as to leave uncovered more or less of the aperture over which it is placed, and admit pure air to mix with and dilute that which has passed through the inhaler. By means of this valve, the vapour may be diluted to any extent, whilst, at the same time, one may have a knowledge of the strength of the

---

* It is the same face-piece I used in giving ether for three or four months before Dr. Simpson introduced the use of chloroform. By the removal of the peculiar expiratory valve, which is its most important part, and the introduction of a sponge, it has been made to constitute a chloroform inhaler by more than one practitioner. These inhalers are, undoubtedly, better than the sponge or handkerchief; but, besides the want of affording due command over the strength of the vapour, I consider that they are open to objection from the chloroform being so near to the mouth, that some of it might be inhaled, by a forcible inspiration, in the form of minute drops, when it would cause temporary spasm of the glottis.

vapour the patient is breathing; not exact, to be sure, but practically of great value. The valves in this face-piece act properly, and close of themselves, in every position in which a patient can be placed, except on his face, and even in this posture they will act if the head be turned on one side.

The position of the patient and inhaler have nothing to do with the specific gravity of the vapour, as some have supposed. If what the patient breathes were as heavy as the pure vapour, it would impose no appreciable labour on the muscles of respiration to raise it to the mouth; and although the vapour of chloroform is four times as heavy as atmospheric air, it does not increase the specific gravity of the air the patient inhales by more than one-fourth; and, indeed, air charged with vapour of chloroform is not so heavy as when charged with vapour of ether at the same temperature. The most convenient position of the patient taking chloroform is lying on the back or side, with the head and shoulders a little raised, as he is then duly supported in the state of insensibility, and can be more easily controlled if he shall struggle whilst becoming insensible. But there is no objection to the sitting posture, when that is most convenient to the operator.

In the next paper, I shall enter on the details necessary to be observed in giving chloroform in different kinds of surgical operations.

ON

NARCOTISM

BY THE

INHALATION OF VAPOURS.

BY

JOHN SNOW, M.D.

LICENTIATE OF THE ROYAL COLLEGE OF PHYSICIANS.

PARTS EIGHT TO SIXTEEN,

From the London Medical Gazette for 1848, 1849, 1850, *and* 1851.

LONDON:

PRINTED BY WILSON AND OGILVY,

57, SKINNER STREET, SNOWHILL.

1851.

CONTENTS.

~~~~~~~~~~~~~~

ON

NARCOTISM BY THE INHALATION OF VAPOURS.

PART VIII.

Conditions of the patient which influence the action of chloroform — age—strength or debility—hysteria—epilepsy—renal convulsions—pregnancy—disease of the lungs—of the heart—tendency to congestion of the brain—diet previously to inhaling—Administration of chloroform in amputations.

BEFORE entering further on the subject of the administration of chloroform, it will be expedient to inquire what are the circumstances, if any, which forbid its use. And experience requires me to make the remark of this substance, which I made last year of ether,—that I know of no state of the patient, with respect either to age, constitution, or disease, which positively contraindicates the use of it, where it is required to prevent the pain of a severe operation, or, I may add, of one the patient greatly dreads. In making this statement, I must not be considered to be recommending the indiscriminate use of chloroform. On the contrary, I consider that everything connected with the patient should be taken into the account, and duly weighed, and the decision arrived at accordingly. And when I state that I have administered chloroform in almost every possible condition in which a patient could require an operation, it must not be considered that I have acted without discrimination, but rather, that going on gradually, and acting on previous experience, supposed objections have one by one vanished, and it has appeared that care in the mode of giving the vapour was the main guarantee, both of safety and success. This view of the subject is entertained by others as well as myself; for, it must be recollected, that I have never given chloroform or ether in an operation, without the concurrence of other medical men.

Chloroform acts more pleasantly, however, on some patients than on others; and we may therefore proceed to consider the circumstances which influence its mode of action. The period of life in which chloroform acts most pleasantly is childhood. In children under thirteen years of age it scarcely ever causes either mental excitement, or any of the struggling which is not unusual in adults just before insensibility ensues, and immunity from pain is obtained with less narcotism of the nervous centres than in older subjects, as I stated before. It is never necessary to carry the narcotism further than the beginning of the third degree in children, at which time I believe their eyes are always turned up; and very often it is not requisite to carry the effects of the vapour beyond the second degree. Indeed, I have seen a child look about it, with a smile on its face, in the middle of the operation of lithotomy.

In a paper which I read at the beginning of the year, I recommended ether for children, in preference to chloroform, on account of the action of the latter being extremely rapid in young patients; but with the apparatus I described in the last paper, the vapour of chloroform can be so diluted with air as to become as mild and gradual in its action as one pleases, and since I have had small face-pieces suited for infants, I have generally given chloroform, and have administered it to a great number of children,

R

[41]

from three weeks old upwards. But when the practitioner is only provided with a handkerchief or sponge, I still consider that the use of chloroform is not perfectly safe, and that ether ought to be employed.

As age advances, the action of chloroform, though equally safe and effectual, is less uniformly pleasant in appearance. In old age, indeed, there is frequently either groaning or a slight degree of stertor, not only during an operation, but even before it begins; so that the effect of the vapour, although quite as satisfactory to the patient, is less agreeable to the friends who may be looking on, than in young subjects. I have often exhibited chloroform in extreme old age, and always with the best effects: indeed, I consider that age is not a source of danger when care is taken. Old people are generally rather longer than others in recovering their consciousness, probably because, owing to their circulation and respiration being less active, the vapour requires a longer time to escape by the lungs. They sometimes do not perfectly recover their former state till twenty minutes or half an hour has elapsed from the conclusion of the operation.

The general condition of the patient as regards robustness, or the contrary, has a considerable influence on the way in which chloroform acts. Usually the more feeble the patient is, whether from illness, or any other cause, the more quietly does he become insensible; whilst if he is strong and robust, there is very likely to be mental excitement in the second degree, and rigidity of the muscles, and probably struggling in the third degree of narcotism. This action of the muscles generally occurs when they are well nourished, whilst in the cases in which they are flaccid, and probably pale, it is usually absent.

The special conditions termed diatheses, seem to have no regular influence over the action of chloroform, except the hysterical one, and this is apt to occasion a little trouble; for as soon as a patient who is subject to hysteria loses her consciousness, from the effect of the vapour, a paroxysm of the complaint is sometimes occasioned. This, however, can always be subdued by proceeding with the inhalation. But the hysterical state, in a few in-

stances, returns, and becomes troublesome, as the effect of the vapour subsides. In two cases that I have met with, it continued for three or four hours. I saw one case, indeed, in which the hysteria lasted much longer, but it was kept up by the alarm of the practitioner in attendance, who was not well acquainted with the action of chloroform,—had given, I believe, an overdose in the first instance, and afterwards mistook the hysteria for the continued effect of the vapour. I was called upwards of thirty hours after the inhalation, when the anxious attendance on the young woman being discontinued, and some of the usual remedies for hysteria applied, she began to amend, but remained in indifferent health for some time. I believe that one or two cases of continued convulsions after chloroform and ether, related in the medical journals, were cases of hysteria. In trying to estimate how far the provocation of hysteria is a drawback from the benefits of chloroform, it must be remembered that the pain of an operation, and still more, perhaps, the anticipation of it, would cause an attack of hysteria in many patients; and I think the proper view to take of the subject is, that whilst a tendency to this complaint ought strictly to forbid the inhalation for amusement, which was at one time somewhat the fashion, it should not interfere with its use in a painful operation, or in any necessary operation, to which the patient cannot otherwise be induced to submit.

Persons subject to epilepsy are liable to have a fit brought on by inhaling ether or chloroform. This occurred in a young lady who had a tumor of the lower jaw removed by the late Mr. Liston, and took ether, but I was able to subdue the convulsions before the operation began, by continuing the vapour, and with chloroform, this, of course, could be more quickly accomplished. It was stated, in one of the foreign medical journals, that chloroform is so certain to cause a fit in epileptic persons, that it may be used to detect impostors pretending to be subject to this disease; but Dr. Todd, who has used chloroform with some advantage in the treatment of epilepsy, in King's College Hospital, has informed me that it does not always produce an attack, even when carried to the extent of causing complete insensibility.

I may here mention a case, though not connected with a surgical operation, in which chloroform caused a recurrence of renal convulsions, from which the patient had been suffering:—A working man, aged about 35, had been in ill health for some weeks before I was called to him on Feb. 19, on account of his being found insensible on the floor. He had in some measure recovered when I arrived, but was in a state of partial stupor, which on the following day was increased, and accompanied with violent convulsions. There was œdema of the face and extremities, and his urine was albuminous, scanty, and of diminished specific gravity. He was bled from the arm, and took digitalis and potash, and on the 22nd, had quite recovered from the convulsions and stupor, and the urine was improved. On the 23rd, however, he became affected with delirium cum tremore, and in the evening I administered chloroform to him, having seen it apparently of service in two or three cases of this disorder. It no sooner began to take effect, however, than violent convulsions came on, of exactly the same kind as those with which he had been affected three days before, and accompanied with the same frightful distortion of the features. Although I did not deem it unsafe to continue the chloroform, I thought it more advisable to discontinue it, and to try the effect of opium. The chloroform having been left off, the convulsions almost immediately subsided, and in three or four minutes the patient was in his former state of delirium. He took twenty-five minims of tincture of opium, and the same dose three hours afterwards. He had a good night's rest, the next day was free from the delirium, and he gradually recovered his health. At the time the patient took the chloroform, there is no doubt that his blood still contained a certain amount of urea and other impurities, and the vapour seemed to act as an additional quantity of these impurities would have done, whilst opium had a different and beneficial effect.

Having noticed the general conditions of the patient, it remains to be inquired how far local disease interferes with the action of chloroform; but pre-viously, the state of pregnancy may be noticed. I recollect two instances in which the patients were pregnant. One was that of a lady, about six months advanced, for whom Mr. Rogers removed some teeth. The chloroform had been recommended by her usual physician before I saw her. The other was a patient in St. George's Hospital, less advanced in pregnancy, on whom Mr. H. C. Johnson operated for the removal of a small fatty tumor. The result was quite favourable in both cases. The narcotism was carried only just to the third degree, and I think that care should be taken not to induce very profound insensibility in pregnancy.

Any affection of the lungs that would not prevent a surgical operation, would be no impediment to the administration of chloroform. I have exhibited it in a few cases in which there was evidence of crude tubercles, and in one case in which cavities existed, and the only result was, that the cough was generally relieved for a day or two afterwards. This has generally been the case also in chronic bronchitis, which has existed in a considerable number of patients. There is sometimes a troublesome fit of coughing at the commencement of the inhalation, when any pulmonary affection exists, but this soon subsides. I have not seen the least injury to the respiratory organs result from the use of chloroform in any instance.

I have already alluded to affections of the heart, and have little to remark now, except that chloroform, carefully administered, is less likely to be prejudicial than severe pain. The patients, however, should be attended to afterwards, and if the chloroform is followed by sickness and coldness, as happens in a few cases, warmth should be applied externally, cordials given, and, if necessary, effervescing draughts, or an opiate. Patients with heart disease, it is well known, are unfavourable subjects for operation under any circumstances; and if they become infected with an animal poison during or subsequent to the operation, have but little chance of recovery. A man, who had dilatation and thinning of the heart, took ether last year, in St. George's Hospital, whilst amputation of the leg was performed. He was attacked with sloughing phagedena, then prevalent, and died on the seventh day, in one of the cold fits attending the disease, there being apparently not strength enough in the heart to establish a re-action from the rigor. And in the case of a gentleman who inhaled chloroform this last summer for the removal of a tumor, and became affected with erysipelas and diffuse cellular inflammation, the symptoms took on a peculiarly low type, and he died on the fifth day. After death there were found dilatation of the heart and thinning of its walls.

As narcotics are usually injurious when there is a tendency to congestion of the brain, it was apprehended by many practitioners that ether and chloroform would be unsafe for such patients; probably the transitory nature of the narcotism induced by inhalation, during an operation, is what renders it harmless. At all events, I have met with no ill results, although some of the patients had suffered from attacks of apoplexy, followed for a time by hemiplegia. This was the case in a man aged 66, on whom Mr. Keate operated, in St. George's Hospital, on the 3rd of August last, for the removal of a tumor situated on the thigh.

It is desirable to give some direction respecting the diet of patients about to inhale chloroform, for if it is inhaled immediately after a meal, there is increased liability to vomiting; and, on the other hand, it is not advisable to inhale after a long fast, for when sickness has occurred in this condition, it has been, in some instances, of considerable duration, and accompanied with more than usual depression. The best preparation appears to be a very moderate breakfast or luncheon two or three hours before the inhalation. The operations in the hospitals are usually performed soon after the patient's dinner hour. The most suitable arrangement in these establishments seems to be, that the subjects of operation should have no dinner, but should have a slender lunch during the forenoon; such as a little bread and butter, bread and milk, or gruel.

Chloroform in amputations.

When moving the patient from his bed to the operating table would cause great pain, as in some cases of ulceration of the cartilages of the knee-joint, the chloroform may be administered with advantage, so as to induce insensibility prior to his being moved. In University and King's College Hospitals, I have exhibited chloroform in several cases of this kind, in the wards, previous to the removal of the patient to the operating theatre, and have afterwards given some more of the vapour just before the operation. In St. George's Hospital this has not been required, as patients so situated have been carried to the theatre on their beds. I have sometimes given just enough chloroform or ether to children to produce unconsciousness, merely to prevent the fright they would experience from seeing any of the preparations for an operation.

The position of the patient usually chosen by the surgeon in the larger amputations—that on the back, with the head and shoulders raised—is very convenient for the chloroform. If the sitting posture is preferred for amputations of the upper extremity, it is desirable to have the patient's back well supported, and the legs raised and supported, either on the couch, or another chair; otherwise he will be liable to slide off his seat when insensible. The tourniquet may be put on either before the inhalation, or after insensibility is induced, but, if before, the screw should not be tightened till afterwards. The tourniquet is occasionally applied during the inhalation in the hospital, in order to save time, and then I inform the patient of the nature of what is being done, that he may not be in dread of the premature use of the knife. It is a good plan to let the patient inhale in a comfortable posture, and then to draw him to the edge of the table, when this is required, just before the operation is commenced.

If two fluid drachms of chloroform be put into the inhaler that has been described, they will usually more than suffice to last to the end of the operation. The face-piece should be at first applied with the expiratory valve turned aside, and this valve should be gradually moved over the aperture, more or less quickly, according to the patient's power of inhaling the vapour, without coughing or complaining of its pungency. So long as he is conscious, his feelings should be attended to, and if nervous, he should be encouraged to persevere with the inhalation; but, when no longer conscious, his apparent dislike of the vapour must not prevent its continuance. The majority of patients become quietly insensible without offering any resistance; but, now and then, the patient, on entering the second degree of narcotism, feeling something unusual, and the purpose of it having escaped from his mind, tries to get rid of the apparatus, and it is necessary to hold his hands. Whilst any voluntary motion continues, either in the eyelids or any other part, all that is required is to go on giving the vapour steadily and gradually. It is seldom necessary to close the expiratory opening completely; it is usually sufficient if the valve cover three-fourths of it, and, if the patient breathe deeply, it should not be more than half covered. When voluntary motion is no longer apparent, in order to become informed respecting the state of the patient, the eyelid should be gently raised, touching its free border. If he look up, it is evident that the narcotism has not exceeded the second degree. If no voluntary motion be excited, the third degree is probably attained, and if the eye be found turned up, this is pretty certain. But, notwithstanding this, if involuntary winking be occasioned by touching the edge of the eyelid, it is necessary to continue the vapour a little longer before the operation is commenced. In doing so, however, if the narcotism have already reached the third degree, and there be no particular rigidity or struggling, the valve may be opened a little further, so as to give the vapour in a more diluted form, or the inhalation may be intermitted for two or three inspirations at a time. In this way, insensibility of the nerves is obtained, without increasing the narcotism of the nervous centres. As soon as the sensibility of the conjunctiva is abolished, or so far blunted that the free edge of the eyelid, or the eye itself, can be touched without causing decided winking, the operation may be commenced with confidence that there will be no pain, and no involuntary flinching that will interfere with the operation. When there is struggling, or great rigidity, in the third degree of narcotism, it is requisite to continue the vapour a little longer till it subside. If there be any

approach to stertorous breathing, the inhalation should at once be suspended, as was stated in a former paper. Stertor, however, never begins till the patient is perfectly insensible. The time occupied in the inhalation is usually from two to three minutes. The operation having been commenced, the medical man having charge of the chloroform should watch the patient's countenance, and if there be any sign of returning sensibility, give a little more vapour during the short time occupied in removing the limb. After the amputation is completed, the vapour need not be repeated until there is decided evidence of sensation. When the arteries to be tied are not numerous, it is sometimes not necessary to repeat the inhalation. Generally, however, it is requisite to give a little chloroform at intervals, and if cold water have to be applied to stop the oozing of blood, or the flaps have to be united by sutures, it is advisable to keep the patient partially insensible till this is done.

———

PART IX.

1. *Condition of patients subsequent to amputation under chloroform.* 2. *They are not more liable to secondary hæmorrhage.* 3. *Statistics of result of amputations under ether and chloroform.* 4. *Their administration in minor amputations.* 5. *In lithotomy.* 6. *Results of cases of lithotomy.* 7. *Chloroform in lithotrity.* 8. *In the treatment of stricture.* 9. *In operation for necrosis.* 10. *In the removal of tumors of the female breast.* 11. *In the removal of tumors of the maxillary bones, and other large operations on the face.*

1. IN amputations under chloroform, the patient is not only saved the immediate pain of the operation, but generally, also, the greater part of the subsequent smarting; for the common sensibility usually remains more or less blunted for some time after the return of consciousness, and the smarting is often not felt at all for half an hour after the operation, and then but slightly. In a few cases, however, pain is felt in the wound as soon as consciousness returns. In two or three cases in which the smarting was dis-

tressing, I have exhibited a little chloroform, from time to time, with complete relief, during the first hour or two that followed the operation; after which the pain shewed no tendency to return. I have tried the local application of chloroform, over the wound, in one or two instances, but it was applied external to other dressings, and not much effect was observed from it. The nervous system is tranquillized by the chloroform inhaled during amputations, and the spasmodic starting of the stump, that without its use would generally be distressing, hardly ever occurs.

2. One of the reports in circulation, soon after the inhalation of ether was introduced, was, that it gave rise to secondary hæmorrhage—probably some surgeon met with it in one or two cases. Secondary hæmorrhage, however, is by no means common after either chloroform or ether. Although I have administered one or other of these vapours in fifty-seven cases of the larger amputations, there has not been secondary hæmorrhage of any consequence, except in two instances, and it has been equally uncommon after other operations. As inhalation prevents the fainting that would otherwise often attend an operation, and generally also stimulates the circulation more or less, we might expect that it would facilitate the tying of all the vessels, and thus be a means of preventing secondary hæmorrhage; and experience seems to confirm this view.

3. Preventing the severe pain of the larger operations may reasonably be supposed to have some effect in diminishing their danger; and as the result of the larger amputations had previously been made the subject of statistical inquiry, they at once suggest themselves as a means of comparing the present with former practice. But a statistical inquiry is evidently incapable of shewing what is the direct effect of the use of chloroform and ether on the mortality resulting from operations. For, if a slight difference should be found, it might be supposed to depend on the altered circumstances under which operations are sometimes performed since the introduction of anæsthetics; as, on the one hand, patients are occasionally induced to submit to them earlier, and when the circumstances are

more favourable than they otherwise would be; and, on the other hand, an amputation is now and then undertaken, when the patient is so reduced, or his prospect of recovery from it so bad, that it would not performed if the pain had to be inflicted. Still, it is proper to make a statistical inquiry, as it would be interesting to know whether the use of those agents has any appreciable effect, direct or indirect, on the mortality; and it may assist to dispel the fears of those, if any such remain, who think that the inhalation of them would be attended with notable ill consequences. With this view, I will here give the result of all the large amputations in which I have administered chloroform or ether. Although the number of cases I have to furnish is not large enough to determine this question, it will serve as a contribution towards that object.

The amputations in which ether was the substance employed, were 32 in number, and took place in 1847; those with chloroform were 25. Of these 57 amputations, five occurred in private practice; three of the thigh, of which two ended fatally; one of the leg, and one of the arm, both followed by recovery; 39 were performed in St. George's Hospital; 22 were amputations of the thigh, amongst which were six deaths; 13 of the leg, followed by three deaths; two of the arm, with one death; and two of the fore-arm, both ending in recovery. Eight of the amputations took place in University College Hospital; five of the thigh, all ending in recovery; two of the leg, in one of which the patient died; and one of the arm, which terminated fatally. Four amputations of the thigh occurred in King's College Hospital, with one death; and there was one amputation of the leg in the Hospital of the Fusilier Guards, performed by Mr. Judd: the patient recovered. The deaths were each occasioned by some well-recognised cause, which the inhalation could neither induce nor prevent: generally erysipelas or inflammation of the veins.

The following table shews the result of all these cases together. None of them remain under treatment; and all the patients who did not actually recover, are included in the deaths, by whatever cause decease was occasioned:

Seat of Amputation.	No. of Cases.	No. of Recoveries.	No. of Deaths.	Deaths per cent.
Thigh	34	25	9	26
Leg	17	13	4	23
Arm	4	2	2	—
Fore-arm	2	2	0	—
Total	57	42	15	26

If the two cases of amputation of the fore-arm be withdrawn, the total mortality will be 27 per cent. instead of 26. None of the above amputations were performed immediately after an accident, but were all either for disease or injuries sustained some time previously.* The mortality in the above cases is a little higher than shewn in a return by Dr. Lawrie of the amputations (primary ones being excluded) at the Glasgow hospital a few years ago,† but is much lower than a similar return by Prof. Malgaigne, from the Parisian hospitals.‡

In a collection of cases of amputation, from various hospitals, under ether and chloroform, in the Monthly Journal of Medical Science, April 1848, by Dr. Simpson, the mortality appeared much lower than in any previous tables ; but as Dr. Simpson gave no instructions in his application for the return of amputations, that cases still under treatment should be excluded, there is reason to apprehend that he may have included such cases in his table, some of which may have since ended fatally. The return I furnished to him of operations under ether at St. George's Hospital is not correctly inserted in his table. Against the seven cases of amputation of the leg, there is a cypher in the column for deaths, where the number 1 ought to stand. This death arose from sloughing phagedena of the stump. I conclude that the discrepancy was occasioned by some mistake, and that, as I have mentioned it to Dr. Simpson, it will be corrected in his future tables ; for I cannot suppose that it was intentionally withdrawn from the deaths, on account of the disease under which the patient succumbed.

4. In amputations at the ankle-joint, or tarsus, it is of course as needful to give chloroform as when the limb is divided higher up. Amputation of a finger or toe is an operation in which it is generally very desirable to inhale the vapour, as the pain of an amputation by no means diminishes in the same proportion as the size of the part on which it is performed. No particular directions are required respecting the mode of giving chloroform in the minor amputations, as what I have said concerning the larger ones is equally applicable to them.

5. Lithotomy is an operation in which I believe that every surgeon now considers it desirable, if not almost a duty, to have his patient made insensible. The practice of tying the hands and feet together with a bandage, to retain the patient in the required position, is still very properly resorted to. It is better to give the chloroform, so as to remove consciousness, before either the bandaging or introduction of the sound. This is especially desirable in the cases of children, and it is also the best plan in adults, as they begin the inhalation more at their ease. During the bandaging and sounding the effect of the vapour partially goes off, and therefore the inhalation must be resumed for a short time, so as to insure complete insensibility when the incision is made. The symptoms of insensibility were described in the last paper treating of the larger amputations. The patient should not be allowed to recover either consciousness or sensibility till the operation is completed by the extraction of the stone ; and therefore, except when the operation is concluded in an unusually short time, it is necessary to give a little vapour from time to time, whenever the eyes shew that the patient is about to wake, or any slight shrinking or moaning indicates the beginning of

* There have been eight amputations in St. George's Hospital performed immediately after injuries, in which ether or chloroform has been administered by one of the resident medical officers. Five of the patients recovered, two died, and one remains under treatment, going on favourably.
† Med. Gaz. vol. xxvii. p. 394.
‡ Archiv. Gén. de Médicine, tom. lviii. p. 40.

uneasy sensations. It must not be supposed when there are obscure indications of sensation from time to time during an operation, that there is severe pain of which the patient is unconscious, for the truth is, that sensibility returns gradually, as we learn, by actual observation, in those cases where complete consciousness returns before the common sensibity. Under these circumstances, the patient, when first beginning to feel, describes as something pricking or pinching, measures that would without anæsthesia cause intense pain, and does not yet feel what at another time would be attended with considerable suffering.

6. The cases of lithotomy, in which I have administered ether or chloroform, are nineteen in number, of which fourteen ended in recovery, and five in death. Eight of the operations were performed in St. George's Hospital, the patients being all children. They all recovered but one, and in that case there was extensive disease of the bladder and kidneys, one of which was dilated so as to form a pouch. Five of the cases occurred in University College Hospital, under the late Mr. Liston; two of the patients were children, and recovered; three were adults, of whom two recovered, and one—a very old man—died. Two of the cases were in King's College Hospital, both in children, and ended in recovery. And there have been four cases in private practice, all those of adults, three of whom died a few days after the operation, and one recovered. The three patients who died were far advanced in life, and their disease was of long standing. The patient who recovered could not have got through the operation had it not been for the chloroform : such was the opinion of Sir B. Brodie and Mr. Coulson. I alluded to this case in a paper I read last winter.*

It will be observed that twelve of the above cases were those of children, and that all of them recovered but one, who had a mortal disease at the time of operation ; and that of the seven adults, four died. This difference between the mortality of lithotomy in childhood, and in the later periods of life, is in accordance with the usual experience of surgeons. I may remark of the cases that were fatal, that death was

* Lancet, Feb. 12, 1848.

the result of causes quite independent of the narcotic vapour, as in all the other cases that I have seen in which operations have ended unfavourably.

7. Chloroform is generally given in St. George's Hospital in lithotrity. As the pain of this operation is usually not excessive, inhalation would not be employed if the surgeons did not feel quite satisfied of its perfect safety, and freedom from all ill effects. I have always seen the operation very satisfactorily performed under chloroform, both in this hospital, and on two occasions when I assisted Mr. Henry Chas. Johnson with it, in private practice. Besides preventing what pain there would be, the surgeons find that the chloroform has the further advantages of preventing the straining efforts of the patient, and enabling them to seize and crush more fragments at one operation than they otherwise could.

The chief suffering from lithotrity is often in passing the fragments ; and in dismissing this subject I may allude to the opinion of the late Mr. Liston, expressed to his class in 1847, that the discovery of etherization would be a reason for choosing lithotomy in some cases, where otherwise crushing the calculus would be preferred, as the former operation at once frees the bladder from irritation, and is now stript of its greatest terror.

8. In the division of the urethra in the perineum, chloroform or ether is of course as necessary as in lithotomy. I have assisted with the inhalation in several such operations. One case may be alluded to here, on account of its important bearing on the treatment of stricture. It was a case in which this operation was about to be performed by Mr. Liston in University College Hospital, but was not required, owing to the relaxing effects of ether on the stricture.

John Willis, aged 42, had stricture of the urethra, caused by an injury twelve years before. He had passed his urine in a very small stream for the last three years, and latterly only by drops, and no catheter could be introduced, although it had been frequently attempted. When the patient was got fully under the influence of ether, a Number 1 catheter was introduced with the intention of passing it down to the stricture, preparatory to dividing it, by an incision in the middle line of the perineum; but it passed right on into the bladder, and the intended operation was not required. This took place on June 18, 1847; the catheter was retained in the bladder till the 23rd, when No. 2 was substituted for it, and subsequently larger catheters, and the patient went out cured on July 27th, being able to pass his urine in a good stream.

9. There are no operations in which the utility of narcotic vapours is greater than in those for necrosis—operations that are generally of considerable duration, and which are amongst the most painful in surgery, on account of the great sensibility of the inflamed bone surrounding the sequestrum. I have given ether and chloroform in nearly thirty operations for necrosis in St. George's Hospital, besides a number elsewhere. The action of the vapour has always been quite effectual in preventing the pain. The majority of the patients were children, and during a great part of the time occupied in the operation narcotism generally did not exceed the second degree; that is to say, there was a dreaming or wandering condition of the mind, and not a state resembling coma.

10. The extirpation of tumors is perhaps the most frequent operation in surgery; but tumors differ so much in size, situation, and every other respect, that there would be no advantage in stating the general result of their removal. Operations for the excision of tumors of the female breast, however, sufficiently resemble each other to admit of such a statement being given.

The number of cases in which I have had to give ether or chloroform, for the removal of tumors of the female breast, involving the gland, is thirty-four. Nineteen of them were in private practice, in seventeen of which the patients recovered from the operation, and in two cases the patients died—one of them of pleurisy, and the other, apparently, of exhaustion. The other fifteen patients were in St. George's Hospital: thirteen recovered from the operation, and two died—one of peritonitis twenty-four days after the operation, the other of erysipelas.

By far the greater number of these tumors of the breast were of a malignant nature. There has not yet been time to ascertain the ultimate effect of the operation on the disease; and, indeed, I am not able to give the result to the present period. The patients in the hospital leave when they have recovered from the operation, and generally are not heard of again; and I only hear now and then, through their surgeons, of some of those in private practice. I am able, however, to state that some of the patients are now in pretty good health, who must long since have died a lingering and painful death if no operation had been performed. Any objections that existed to the removal of malignant tumors must have been greatly diminished by the introduction of narcotic vapours. Each case must, of course, be judged on its own merits; but the number of cases in which an operation may be properly recommended, and in which it will be submitted to, when the whole question is laid before the patient, must be considerably increased by the discovery of the means of rendering it devoid of pain.

11. The only surgical operations that present any difficulty to the total prevention of pain during their performance, are operations of considerable magnitude and duration, which involve the cavity of the mouth or nose, such as the removal of tumors of the maxillary bones. The patient can be rendered insensible before the operation, in the usual way, as easily as in other cases; but the difficulty is in repeating the inhalation so as to preserve the immunity from pain till its conclusion. It is best, in operations of the face, to exhibit the vapour well diluted, so that insensibility may be induced gradually, by which means the fluids of the body get more thoroughly impregnated, and its effects are more permanent. When inhalation of chloroform extends over three or four minutes, and the third degree of narcotism is well established, with insensibility of the conjunctiva, it is generally about three minutes before there are distinct signs of pain from the use of the knife. The effects of ether are, I think, a little more lasting, and therefore it would be preferable in such operations, were it not that chloroform can be more easily reapplied during the operation. To effect this, I drop a few minims of it, from time to time, on a sponge that has been squeezed out of cold water, and as soon as the patient evinces any sign of pain,

c

I apply it near to his mouth and nostrils for a moment, whenever the position of the surgeon's hands, and those of his assistants, will permit. In this way, if the pain cannot all be prevented, the patient can generally be kept so unconscious that he afterwards says that he felt nothing. It is only in protracted operations that the use of the sponge in this way is required, for the greater number of operations are concluded in two or three minutes.

There are some surgeons who think that chloroform in operations involving the mouth, and attended with considerable hæmorrhage, is not altogether free from the danger of blood getting into the trachea. This point requires to be very carefully considered, for whilst it would be improper to run a risk of this occurrence, the pain of large operations on the face is so frightful that the inhalation ought not to be interdicted on mistaken grounds. There are good physiological reasons for believing that the sensibility of the glottis would last, under the influence of narcotics, as long as respiration continued to be performed; but the best evidence will be that derived from experience. I have seen a great number of operations attended with considerable hæmorrhage into the mouth, in which ether or chloroform has been given, and no ill effects have followed in any case. The result of my observation consequently is, that there is no danger of blood getting into the air passages when these agents are carefully given, and the same attention is paid to the patient's position and breathing that would be in the absence of insensibility. There was one operation at which I assisted last summer, where the patient died soon after it was performed, and as I have heard that a report got abroad, in some parts of the medical world, that death was occasioned by blood entering the air-passages, it may here be mentioned:—

The patient was a young man, with a large fibrous tumor in the situation of the left superior maxillary bone. For some time previous to the operaton he had suffered occasionally from hæmorrhage from the affected nostril, to an extent which had reduced him considerably. The vapour was given to him rather slowly, with the apparatus I commonly employ, and he became gradually insensible, without previous excitement or struggling. In about three minutes the inhalation was discontinued, the narcotism having reached the third degree. The patient was passive, but the muscles were not relaxed. The breathing was not stertorous. Some teeth were now extracted without causing any sign of pain. A little more chloroform was then given to him, and when the inhalation was discontinued a second time he was in the same state as before the teeth were drawn. The operation was immediately commenced. I took no notes of the method in which it was performed, but can state that the superior maxillary and malar bones of the left side were removed. During the first part of the operation, whilst the flaps were made, the patient was perfectly quiet and silent; but afterwards he began to groan and move his limbs, and he was not again rendered altogether insensible; for although a few minims of chloroform were from time to time sprinkled over a sponge, which was, now and then, held near his face, yet, owing to the hands of the operator and his assistants being in the way, and the cavity of the mouth and nostril being laid widely open, he got very little of the vapour, and the only effect of it was partially to quiet him on one or two occasions. After the first two or three minutes of the operation the effect of the chloroform never exceeded the second degree. The patient executed voluntary movements of his arms and legs; sometimes it was necessary to hold his hands, and at one time he appeared conscious, for he folded his arms as if making an effort not to raise his hands to the seat of pain. He coughed now and then, and seemed somewhat embarrassed with the blood in his throat. He was seated in a chair, but as there was no window in the operating theatre except the skylight, his head was obliged to be inclined rather backwards. He was leaned forwards once or twice, to allow him to get rid of the blood, and it appeared that he vomited some on one of these occasions. Towards the conclusion of the operation, and at a time when he was very little under the influence of chloroform, he fainted. He was laid down, and brandy was given to him. No more chloroform was administered after this time. He partially rallied from the syncope, but again became faint. The actual cautery was applied, but oozing of blood continued until the moment of death,—about half an hour after his removal into another room. During this interval he was much exhausted; his pulse was small, and difficult to feel. He was tossing himself about in a restless manner, but there was no difficulty of breathing. He seemed quite conscious, doing as he was told, but, of course, could not speak, from the nature of the operation. I left a few minutes before the patient's death. When he ceased to breathe, tracheotomy was performed, and artificial respiration exercised by the opening, with no beneficial result. In my opinion this measure was not indicated, but of course it could do no harm.

After death, portions of the tumor were found still remaining attached to the posterior and upper part of the cavity, and projecting into the foramen lacerum of the orbit and right nostril, as well as in other directions. The trachea and bronchi contained some frothy blood. Numerous small dark spots of congestion were met with in the lung, resulting from some of the small bronchi being filled with blood.

It is evident that the chloroform did not contribute, either directly or indirectly, to this patient's death, for the following reasons:—1st. That the tracheotomy and artificial respiration sufficiently account for the small quantity of blood found in the bronchial tubes. (An eminent physician-accoucheur has informed me that in cases of still-born children, in which he has performed artificial respiration by an incision in the larynx, he has always found blood, after death, in the bronchi.) 2nd. If there had not been this reason for blood in the lungs, it would be more likely to have entered when the patient was moribund, or during the syncope, than at an earlier period. 3rd. That the symptoms did not indicate any impediment to respiration, but were such as I have seen in uterine hæmorrhage, and such as were met with after the removal of the superior maxillary bone by a very eminent operator in this metropolis, before the introduction of ether. 4th. That if the judicious use of chloroform caused a liability to the entrance of blood into the bronchi, there would have been some symptoms of it in the numerous patients who have recovered from similar operations in the narcotised state; but such is not the case. And 5th. That the quantity of blood met with in the lungs was not enough to cause rapid death.

In dismissing this case, I wish to state my belief that the operation was a very proper endeavour to cure the patient of a disease that must inevitably have been fatal in a short time; and that my reason for alluding to it is, that if I should leave it unnoticed, in treating of chloroform in operations on the face, I might be suspected of keeping back a material fact.

I will now enumerate the other operations, for the removal of larger tumors of the jaw, in which I have exhibited narcotic vapours.

In May 1847, Mr. Liston removed a large tumor of the lower jaw, in a young lady, dividing the bone far back, near the rami, on each side. He was assisted by Mr. Morton, Mr. Cadge, and others. The patient took ether.

On December 23, 1847, Mr. Henry Charles Johnson removed one of the superior maxillary bones of a young man, in St. George's Hospital, for a large tumor. This, and the remaining patients, inhaled chloroform.

A few days after the last operation, Mr. Fergusson removed a large tumor of the lower jaw, occurring in a gentleman. Sir B. Brodie was present.

Early in January 1848, Mr. Fergusson also removed a large tumor of the upper jaw of a middle-aged woman, in King's College Hospital. The tumor had been removed once before, but had returned.

In May last, Mr. Tatum removed a very large tumor of the lower jaw of a Spanish gentleman, in St. George's Hospital, dividing the bone near its symphisis, and disarticulating it on one side.

In November last, Mr. Fergusson removed a tumor of the superior maxillary bone in a little girl, in King's College Hospital.

In the same month, Mr. Fergusson also removed a tumor of the lower jaw in a young man, a patient in the same hospital.

The above patients all recovered favourably from the operation.

I have seen chloroform and ether employed, also, in a number of other operations in which a good deal of blood flows into the mouth and throat; such as operations for epulis, and polypi of the nose. Sometimes the patients can be observed to swallow the blood, with an act of deglutition; but usually it seems to flow down the pharynx and œsophagus without distinct muscular effort; and if the quantity of it is not very large, it does not in any way interfere with the glottis.

When infants are laid on the back, during the operation for hare-lip, the blood is swallowed, whether they are narcotised or not; and when they are insensible, it goes down with less appearance of choking than when they are crying from pain.

———

PART X.

1. *Ether and Chloroform in operations on the teeth; 2 on the eye; 3. on the anus; 4. on the back. 5. Inhalation to facilitate the reduction of hernia; 6. of dislocations; 7. to aid diagnosis; 8. to save the moral feelings of the patient. 9. Occasional sequelæ of inhalation—sickness; 10. its treatment. 11. Headache. 12. Hysteria.*

1. CHLOROFORM is, I believe, not very generally employed in tooth-drawing in this metropolis. This is partly owing to the circumstance, that the pain occasioned by the operation, though severe, is usually but momentary; but another reason appears to be, that the majority of dentists are not sufficiently acquainted with the application of the medicine to be satisfied that they can use it with perfect safety, and it is not always convenient to the patient to have another medical man present. It is only in the cases of children and very nervous persons, who have not resolution to keep the mouth voluntarily open for the operation, that narcotism facilitates the work of the dentist; in other cases it adds to his trouble, and occupies more of his time. The introduction of ether and chloroform has been of service to the dental profession, having increased the practice of many of its members, by relieving the springs of industry from the incubus of the dread of pain; for a number of the operations under these vapours would not have been performed except for their use. I allude to many of the cases in which the mouth is "cleared," as the term is,

of a number of decayed teeth, and stumps of teeth, to make room for a set of artificial ones—a process which is now generally performed at one or two sittings, without any pain, and which cannot fail to be, ultimately, of great benefit to the patients.

It is desirable not to carry the narcotism further than the third degree for the extraction of teeth, and in this stage there is generally some rigidity of the muscles of the jaw, but this can nearly always be overcome by pressing the chin down. It has been recommended that a wedge should be placed in the mouth before the inhalation, but I have never seen it necessary to have recourse to this plan, as I have always been able, with the assistance of the operator, to get the patient's mouth open. The few instances in which the mouth could not be at once opened were cases in which voluntary power was exerted under a dreaming condition of the mind, and in these cases the exhibition of a little more of the vapour enabled the desired object to be effected. There was one instance in which the addition to the dose of vapour was prevented by hysterical symptoms, till the lady recovered her consciousness, and then she had sufficient courage, and preferred to have her tooth removed without the repetition of the inhalation, which there is no doubt would have been effectual, as in every other case that I have seen. As it was, the pain was probably diminished. It has always appeared to me that there was a diminution of muscular power under the effects of chloroform and ether, in every variety of their operation; the voluntary efforts under excitement are much less powerful than those of an exasperated individual in an unnarcotised state, and the involuntary rigidity in the third degree is still more easily overcome. As there is usually less rigidity from the use of ether than chloroform, the former would be preferable in tooth-drawing, were it not for the strong odour that it leaves in the breath for the rest of the day. When teeth require to be removed from both jaws, those in the lower one, especially if they be molars, should be first extracted; otherwise, as the patient is unable to wash out his mouth, the blood will render them obscure. To clear the mouth of blood, whilst operating on the teeth of the lower jaw, it is sometimes desirable to use a sponge squeezed out of warm water. If the sensibility is found to be returning before all the teeth are extracted, the inhalation must be resumed for a short time before proceeding further. There is sickness after the use of chloroform in some instances of dental as of other operations, and it is here felt to be more annoying than after a great operation where the patient is necessarily an invalid. I shall have to speak of the treatment of sickness further on.

I am not an advocate for the use of chloroform in every instance of tooth-drawing, but I do not see how any rules can be laid down respecting its employment, as a good deal must depend on the wishes of the patient as well as on the presumed severity of the operation. One point, however, should be imperative, viz. that chloroform should not be given except by medical men who have made themselves well acquainted with its effects and mode of application. I have a strong feeling that severe pain ought not to be inflicted on children, since the means of preventing it have been discovered, and act so favourably on them; and therefore, when a tooth is to be removed that is firmly fixed, I think that a child should be made insensible whenever there is the knowledge requisite to effect this with perfect safety.

2. In most operations on the eye, narcotism is of essential service. In the operation for strabismus, the amount of pain to be prevented is considerable; and as the patients are usually children, who would offer all the resistance in their power, the proceedings of the surgeon are very much facilitated, as Prof. Miller, of Edinburgh, has recently remarked.* Chloroform or ether may be given with advantage to children, in operations on the eye unattended with pain, merely for the purpose of keeping the patient and the eye motionless. I have given the vapour of one or other of these medicines several times for Mr. Cæsar Hawkins and Mr. George Pollock, whilst operating on congenital cataract by the method of drilling. Two or or three of the latter gentleman's pa-

* Surgical Experience of Chloroform.

tients were only a few weeks old. The operation was facilitated in all the cases. In the excision of cataract, it is not advisable to administer ether or chloroform, for if vomiting should be induced it would be likely to cause serious mischief; and although vomiting is not a frequent result of inhalation, when precautions are taken to prevent it, yet it is impossible, I believe, to predict with certainty in any case that it will not occur.

3. Operations on the anus are frequently required, and they are of a very painful nature, on account of the great sensibility of the part. It was the practice of most surgeons before the introduction of inhalation, to have the patient standing on the floor, in a stooping posture, and leaning over a table or bed; but this attitude could scarcely be maintained in a state of insensibility, and therefore the practice now is to let the patient lie on his side, with the knees drawn up towards the abdomen; or when that is more convenient to the surgeon, the patient can lie on his back, as for lithotomy. The chief operations on the anus are that for fistula, the excision of hæmorrhoids, and the cutting away of loose folds of integument from the verge of the anus, for the cure of prolapsus. It is necessary to have the patient completely insensible in operations on this part, more especially in that for fistula, as any involuntary flinching during its performance would be a serious inconvenience.

4. For the removal of tumors from the back, and the performance of any other operations in that situation, it is best to let the patient inhale whilst lying on his side, and when he is insensible to turn him over, in a great measure, on his abdomen, allowing his head to remain in its former position on the pillow: in this way the inhalation can be repeated, if required, during the operation.

It is unnecessary to enumerate other operations, as they do not require any special directions, as regards the chloroform or ether. There are some cases to be mentioned, however, in which narcotism is attended with signal benefits, in addition to the prevention of pain.

5. There have been several cases of strangulated hernia, in which the inhalation of ether or chloroform has

enabled the bowel to be replaced by the taxis, after previous efforts had failed, and where an operation must otherwise have been performed. I am not aware how soon etherization was employed with this happy result, but the earliest case that I find recorded is that of a patient of Mr. White in the General Hospital, near Nottingham: it occurred on March 22nd, 1847, and the ether was administered by Dr. Sibson.* On July 10, 1847, there was a similar case under the care of Mr. Stafford, in the Marylebone Infirmary.† On March 6th, 1848, a man, James S., was placed upon the operating table, in St. George's Hospital, with a strangulated inguinal hernia: I administered chloroform to him at the request of Mr. H. C. Johnson, who had the treatment of the case; and when the patient became completely insensible, and the muscular system relaxed, the hernia was readily reduced by means of the taxis, although it was previously quite incapable of reduction. If the taxis had not been successful, the operation, for which the instruments were arranged ready, would at once have been performed, whilst the patient was still insensible. In the case of another patient, a woman with femoral hernia, who was placed on the table immediately afterwards, Mr. Johnson performed the operation as soon as she was rendered insensible, without employing the taxis, being deterred by the tense and inflamed condition of the tumor. This case ended favourably, as well as the former one. There are several other cases recorded in the medical journals of this and other countries, besides the three above enumerated, in which the use of ether or chloroform has enabled the surgeon to reduce a strangulated hernia without the operation.

6. Narcotism by inhalation facilitates the reduction of dislocations of the bones, besides preventing the pain of the process; and it has enabled the surgeon to reduce dislocations of long standing, which could not otherwise have been relieved. On June 24, 1847, Mr. Tatum reduced a dislocation of the shoulder of ten weeks' standing, with the aid of the pullies, in St. George's Hospital, whilst the patient, Richard R., aged 31, was under the influence of ether.

The dislocation, which happened in the country, had been first overlooked, and when detected, could not be reduced. On February 7th, 1848, a dislocation of the femur into the ischiatic notch, which had existed for about three weeks, was reduced with the aid of the pullies, in the same hospital, by Mr. H. C. Johnson; the patient, Patrick C., an Irish labourer, being made insensible, and his muscles being relaxed, with chloroform. Three days afterwards, Mr. Tatum reduced a dislocation of the hip, in the hospital, of five weeks' standing; the patient, Joseph G., a working man, being put under the influence of chloroform. I have also given the vapour, in St. George's Hospital, in some cases of old dislocation, in which the position of the parts has been improved by the efforts made during the state of insensibility and relaxation, although their condition did not admit of complete reduction: two cases of dislocation at the elbow-joint were of this nature. Some cases of recent dislocation have been reduced under the influence of narcotic vapours, when previous attempts at reduction had been unsuccessful. Two cases of dislocation of the thigh-bone, in which Dr. Sibson administered ether, at Nottingham, were of this nature. One into the ischiatic notch, reduced by Mr. White, April 7th, 1847; the other on the dorsum ilii, reduced by Mr. Caunt, May 31st, 1847.* I assisted Mr. H. C. Johnson by giving chloroform to a gentleman with a recent compound dislocation of the last phalanx of the thumb backwards. The previous efforts at its reduction had failed, on account of the pain occasioned by them being more than the patient could bear. When he was rendered insensible, the dislocation was soon reduced.

Chloroform was given in many of the above cases because it was in use at the time, and could be employed without the delay that getting the ether ready would have occasioned. It answered very well; but it is my opinion that ether is preferable, both in dislocations and strangulated herniæ, as it induces relaxation of the muscles more easily, and with less previous rigidity.

7. The artificial production of insensibility is frequently of the utmost service in assisting the surgeon to form

* See MED. GAZ. Vol. xl. p. 1009.
† MED. GAZ. Vol. xl. p. 115.

* See MED. GAZ. Vol. xl. p. 1009.

a diagnosis. I gave ether for this purpose at the request of the surgeons to St. George's Hospital, in February, 1847, to a little girl with disease of the knee and abscesses in the thigh. In this case, the great tenderness of the parts, and the nervous agitation of the patient, precluded every attempt to examine the state of the limb in the usual manner ; but when the patient was rendered insensible, the condition of the limb was ascertained sufficiently to enable the surgeon to determine on amputation, which was performed on February 25th, by Mr. Henry James Johnson, the patient being again placed under the influence of ether. In several other cases of diseased joint and diseased bone, ether and chloroform have been employed in this hospital, to aid diagnosis in a similar manner. In sounding for stone, especially in children, it is of service to render the patient unconscious. I administered ether for this purpose in St. George's Hospital, as early as February 3rd, 1847, whilst Mr. Cutler sounded a little boy, aged four years. Dr. Thomas Smith, of Cheltenham, applied ether about this time, viz. on February 22nd, to enable him to ascertain the state of the corneæ of a child labouring under strumous ophthalmia.*

8. There are many operations on the female which medical students could seldom witness except at the expense of some shock to the feelings of the patient. They are now generally conducted in the hospitals in this wise :— The patient inhales and becomes insensible whilst only one or two surgeons and the nurse are present in the private ward, or behind the screen with her : the students then come in and witness the operation, and go away again before the consciousness of the patient has returned. In some operations in private practice, where the surgeon requires two or three assistants, they are not brought into the room till the patient is insensible, or she is made insensible in an adjoining room, and carried to the place selected for the operation.

9. Narcotism by chloroform or ether, to the extent required in surgical operations, occasionally leaves some effects after the immediate influence of the vapour has subsided : these may be called sequelæ. I have not observed that they are more frequent after one of these agents than the other. The only after-effects of inhalation with which I am acquainted are sickness, headache, and hysterical symptoms in those predisposed to hysteria.

Vomiting is apt to occur during the narcotism, or just afterwards. It can be rendered less frequent by the precaution previously mentioned,* of not allowing the patient to inhale soon after a meal, and also not carrying the narcotism further, if possible, than the third degree,—thus avoiding stertor and complete relaxation of the muscular system ; but I believe that it cannot always be prevented by all the care that can be used, more especially if the inhalation have to be repeated, in order to keep up the insensibility for more than a few minutes. The vomiting no doubt depends on the action of the narcotic vapour on the brain, and is allied to that occasionally caused by opium and alcohol, and to that which occurs in some morbid conditions of the cerebrum. If the patient recover completely from the immediate effects of the vapour, without any feeling of sickness, he is not liable to it afterwards from that cause; and, in the greater number of cases in which vomiting does occur, the sickness goes off in a few minutes, and does not return ; but in a few instances it continues for several hours, if nothing be done to relieve it, and in two or three cases it has lasted, under these circumstances, for two or three days. I have met with more or less vomiting in about one-fifth of the patients operated on, under chloroform, during the last six months : many of them, however, had received no previous directions respecting their diet. The number of cases in which there has been troublesome sickness has been one in twenty-six operations during the same period. I have never found the sickness continue more than five or six hours when I have been taking measures to relieve it.

Diminished temperature of the surface generally accompanies the sickness : indeed, the depression of the respiration and circulation attending it has a tendency at all times to lessen the development of animal heat. But

---

* See MED. GAZ. Vol. xl. p. 676.

* Last vol. p. 1024.

chloroform and ether, I am quite satisfied, have also the effect of diminishing the production of caloric, quite independently of their action on the respiration and circulation; and, when inhalation has been kept up for some time, I have remarked the patient to become rather cold in cases where no sickness was present.

10. When sickness has continued after the immediate effects of the vapour have subsided, and the stomach has been quite emptied by vomiting, I have generally found that a little wine or weak brandy and water has removed the sickness. When the patient is cold as well as sick, warm wine and water, or brandy and water, are preferable; and other measures to restore warmth should be resorted to, such as warm covering, drawing the sofa near the fire, if it be winter, or applying a feet-warmer, if the patient be in bed. In two or three cases these measures did not afford relief, and ten or twelve minims of Battley's solution of opium were given, with the effect of completely and permanently removing the sickness: these, of course, were adult patients, and I have not found sickness continue very long in children. The horizontal posture should, if possible, be preserved till the sickness has subsided, and for some time afterwards. It is desirable, indeed, to let the patient remain, without being moved or spoken to, till the narcotism has completely passed off, in every instance where it is practicable. The necessary removal of hospital patients from the operating theatre immediately after the operation causes sickness in many cases where I believe that it would not otherwise come on. I have not perceived any appreciable benefit from effervescing draughts, and I have not had occasion to try hydrocyanic acid or creosote. The application of ammonia to the nostrils sometimes seems to refresh the patient, but internally I think it is not so beneficial as wine.

The wine and opium recommended above are not given to combat the direct effects of chloroform, and should not be administered till the immediate influence of the vapour has subsided, unless it be the former, when it is required to remove faintness from loss of blood, which, however, seldom happens during narcotism. The opium probably acts by removing irritability of the stomach, occasioned by the vomiting, which was induced in the first instance by the state of the brain.

11. Headache is not a common result of inhalation: the few instances in which I have heard it complained of, occurred in persons in good health and inclined to plethora, and passed off spontaneously.

12. In describing the circumstances that modify the action of narcotic vapours, it was stated* that, in the hysterical diathesis, inhalation was liable to induce a paroxysm of the disorder, which might recur as the narcotism was diminishing. This usually soon subsides, but there are a few cases in which it remains troublesome for two or three hours. I have seen hysteria two or three times in the male, after ether and chloroform, in patients who had previously had the complaint. I have not found it to require any treatment, except in the case mentioned before;† and if it do, it should be treated in the usual way.

My own experience of hysteria, as a sequela of inhalation, is, that it forms no great impediment to its employment. Mr. Tomes,‡ however, has related three cases with which he had been made acquainted, where the disorder was more lasting and troublesome; and one case in which the use of chloroform was followed by worse effects than hysteria, viz. delirium, and subsequently an occasional vacancy in the patient's manner, leading her medical man to forbode insanity, sooner or later. In this last case, however, the patient had an overdose of the vapour, having been "almost pulseless — scarcely breathing," with a ghastly countenance. The chloroform was given by a dentist who evidently did not understand its effects, having first asserted that the lady was "under its full influence," when she, in fact, heard what he said, and then having given an overdose. The case only confirms a maxim, now beginning to be better understood than when chloroform was first suddenly brought into universal notice —viz. that it ought not to be used except by medical men who have studied its effects.

---

* Last vol. p. 1022.
† Loc. cit.
‡ See Review in MED. GAZ., last vol. p. 545.

———

PART XI.

The combination of chloroform and ether—of chloroform and alcohol—Chloric ether—Strong chloric ether—New mode of inhaling vapours.

IT has been shown in former parts of this essay, that the action of chloroform can be rendered perfectly mild and safe by diluting it sufficiently with air. If the properties of this body were such, or if another body could be met with having such properties that the relation between its intrinsic power and its volatility would prevent the air from taking up so much vapour, under the usual circumstance of temperature and pressure, as could enable a patient to get an overdose without ample warning, this would be an advantage; as there would then be no fear of accidents in the hands of medical men, even when not armed with a suitable inhaler, and special experience on the subject. This, however, is not the nature of chloroform, and although there are substances of this character, of which I intend to give a further account, they do not possess, at the same time, all the other convenient and agreeable qualities which would enable them to supersede chloroform in the majority of surgical operations. As the most desirable strength of a volatile narcotic liquid, not requiring great care in its use, is between that of chloroform and that of sulphuric ether, it might be supposed that by mixing the two medicines the desired end would be attained: but such is not the case; they have been so mixed by some practitioners, and I have tried them together, but the result is a combination of the undesirable qualities of both, without any compensating advantage. Ether is about six times as volatile as chloroform—that is to say, if equal measures of each be placed in two evaporating dishes kept side by side, at the same temperature, the ether evaporates in about one-sixth the time of the chloroform; and when the two liquids are mixed, although they then evaporate together, the ether is converted into vapour much more rapidly; and, in whatever proportions they are combined, before the whole is evaporated the last portion of the liquid is nearly all chloroform: the

consequence is that at the commencement of the inhalation the vapour inspired is chiefly ether, and towards the end nearly all chloroform : the patient experiencing the stronger pungency of ether when it is most objectionable, and inhaling the more powerful vapour at the conclusion, when there is the most need to proceed cautiously.

Chloroform was first employed for inhalation in the form of solution in alcohol, in which state it was called chloric ether. Mr. Jacob Bell was, I believe, the first person who exhibited it,* and it was afterwards employed occasionally in St. Bartholomew's Hospital, and in the private practice of Mr. Lawrence. This so-called chloric ether contained from twelve to eighteen per cent. of chloroform. When inhaled it yielded a little vapour of chloroform at the beginning of the process. Each hundred cubic inches of air passing over it, would take up, if saturated at 60°, from one and a half to two cubic inches, mixed with some vapour of spirit, and this was enough to produce insensibility if continued of the same strength, but by the time a third part of the liquid was inhaled, the quantity of vapour given off was reduced to less than half a cubic inch, which is insufficient either to induce or keep up insensibility; and when about half the chloric ether had evaporated, the remainder was reduced to spirit and water, with scarcely a trace of chloroform. Consequently, unless the inhaler were frequently emptied and replenished with fresh ether, insensibility failed to be induced; and under any circumstances the use of this preparation was troublesome and expensive.

In some able and interesting articles recently published in the MEDICAL GAZETTE, Dr. John C. Warren, of Boston, U.S., has recommended a strong chloric ether, containing one part chloroform to two parts alcohol; this would be undoubtedly much more efficient than the ordinary chloric ether; but there is the same kind of irregularity in its effects, as in the case of the weaker preparation. The chloroform evaporates chiefly with the first portion of spirit, and when a little more than half the liquid has been used, the remainder contains very little chloroform, and is, therefore, of no use for inhala-

---

* See Pharm. Journ. Feb. 1847, p. 357.

D

tion, since vapour of alcohol has very little effect.

I had often considered the subject of diluting chloroform with spirit, and since Dr. Warren's papers appeared have given the matter additional attention. I have mixed chloroform in various proportions with alcohol of 92·5 per cent. and ascertained the quantity of vapour the compounds would give off. I have also placed these compounds in a current of air, in imitation of what takes place during inhalation, and by measuring the liquid from time to time, and weighing it in the specific gravity bottle, have been able to calculate the changes of composition which take place as evaporation proceeds. In so doing, a correction was made for the small quantity of water in the spirit, the proportion of which increases as the alcohol evaporates. The following table, which is as accurate as can be made without introducing fractions, shows how the proportion of chloroform decreases when it is mixed with an equal volume of alcohol, or with any other quantity marked in the table. For instance, when the hundred parts are diminished to sixty, they constitute the strong chloric ether of Dr. Warren, and the alterations in that compound are subsequently shown. The fourth column exhibits the quantity of chloroform in the mixed vapour that 100 cubic inches of air would take up, if saturated at 60°. The quantity that 100 cubic inches of air will thus take up from pure chloroform, is fourteen cubic inches.

Chloroform and Alcohol.	Alcohol.	Chloroform.	Cubic Inches of Vapour.
100	50	50	8·1
90	48	42	7·8
80	46	34	7·4
70	43	27	6·8
60	40	20	5·9
50	37	13	4·5
40	33	7	2·1
30	27	3	0·9
20	19½	½	0·0
10	10	0	0·0

Dr. Warren recommends the strong chloric ether, in order to prevent the accidents that have resulted from the too rapid action of chloroform. The quantity of vapour of chloroform that air would take up from this compound would, under the usual circumstances of inhalation, not exceed six per cent. —a proportion which, I believe, would not cause any sudden accident; but unless the person using it have such skill as would enable him to avoid the risk of accident in using chloroform, he would be liable to fail in producing insensibility with its solution in spirit, owing to its rapidly decreasing strength, and the diminishing quantity of vapour that it gives off: indeed, Dr. Warren has himself experienced the irregularity of the action of strong chloric ether, having failed to induce insensibility with it in two or three cases; but he attributes the failure to a defect of susceptibility in the patients, and he advises the resort to chloroform in such cases. This is virtually yielding the point, and incurring in some cases the very risk which the proposed practice is intended to obviate. A case which occurred recently in Westminster, the account of which had not reached America when Dr. Warren's papers were written, shows that an apparent want of susceptibility does not protect the patient from accident. In that case,* a gentleman, who, as I am informed, had many times used chloroform in the same way before, employed half an ounce on a handkerchief without making the man insensible; but, a fresh supply being obtained an hour or two afterwards, the patient got an over-dose, and lost his life, although the quantity used was not greater than on the previous occasion. When chloroform is given in such a way that the strength of the vapour can be regulated, it is found that there is no appreciable difference in the susceptibility to its action, whatever variety there may be in the symptoms induced previous to insensibility, and in the extent to which it is requisite to carry the narcotism in order to obtain relaxation or immunity from pain; and since it has been shown in the first three parts of these papers, that there is a definite rule for the proportion of chloroform and other narcotic vapours in the blood, which applies alike to animals of different classes, it cannot be supposed that any human being could form an excep-

---

* See Lancet, Feb. 24.

tion, since he would have to differ, not only from his own species, but from the animal kingdom in general.

When it is necessary to give chloroform on a sponge, during a surgical operation, it is not a bad plan to use it diluted with spirit, as recommended by Dr. Warren. In two or three recent cases of operation on the face, insensibility having been induced before the operation, by means of the apparatus as usual, it was requisite to employ the sponge to keep the patient insensible during its performance; and I employed a solution of chloroform in spirit, sometimes in equal parts, at other times in the proportion constituting the strong chloric ether. Both preparations answer the purpose very well, and can be employed more freely than undiluted chloroform. I poured, for instance, half a drachm or a drachm on the sponge at once, in these cases, instead of a few minims.

If the strong chloric ether were used exactly as recommended by Dr. Warren, there would, I fear, be danger of accident from a cause independent of the action of the vapour inhaled. An ounce of the medicine is directed to be poured on a sponge only twice the size of an egg, which must thereby be rendered dripping wet, and should the patient be on his back, there would be risk of some drops of the ether being drawn into the glottis, in a liquid form. I have been informed by the operator of a case in which a patient was threatened with suffocation from a drop of chloroform falling into the throat from a sponge, and the solution of it in alcohol is scarcely less irritating, and would undoubtedly cause spasm of the glottis.

It follows from the above considerations, that, as a general rule, there can be no advantage in using a mixture of two or more substances of different volatility, by any ordinary method of inhalation, since the mixture cannot be uniformly introduced into the circulation. If, however, it should hereafter be found that there is any physiological advantage in combining any vapours, they could easily be given together in any uniform proportion, by a method which I have been employing lately for the exhibition of chloroform in cases in which I wished to be more than usually precise, or to gain a more exact experience. This method consists in putting a definite quantity of the liquid to be inhaled into a balloon made of thin membrane, the capacity of which is known, and is not less than two thousand cubic inches, then filling the balloon with air by means of the bellows, and allowing the patient to inhale from it: the expired air being prevented from returning into the balloon, by one of the valves in the face-piece to which it is attached.

PART XII.

Further remarks on Dutch liquid—its chemical constitution — its physical properties—its narcotic power compared with that of chloroform—Cases of its administration in tooth-drawing, in midwifery, in cholera—Conclusions.

IN a former paper* I gave an account of two or three experiments on small animals with Dutch liquid, by which it was shown that its narcotic properties were of a favourable kind, but that it caused inflammation of the lungs. This latter effect, as I have since ascertained, was occasioned by some impurity—probably sulphurous acid gas —in the specimen of Dutch liquid I then used. I made it myself, by getting the olefiant gas and chlorine to combine in a glass globe, as recommended in Fownes' Chemistry. The olefiant gas was passed through sulphuric acid to separate ether and alcohol, but the sulphurous acid was not separated from it, and I endeavoured to separate that and the hydrochloric acid from the products, when formed, by washing it two or three times in water, but did not succeed, as it since appears. On Mr. Nunnelly recommending Dutch liquid for inhalation last February, it occurred to me that neither the specimen which I had made, nor that used by Dr. Simpson, could have been pure. I accordingly made some more in the same manner as before, but washed it in a weak solution of carbonate of soda previous to distilling it from chloride of calcium. I now got a much less pungent substance,—similar, in fact, to that which I have since received from Mr. Morson and Mr. Bullock. On performing some experiments with it, I found that it possessed the properties which I previously described, with the exception of the irritant ones. I in-

* Vol. xlii. p. 331.

haled a little of it myself; but the process of making it being very troublesome and tedious, I had not enough to try its effects in practice till half an ounce was kindly given to me by Mr. Morson on the 20th March, which I used in four cases of tooth-drawing in St. George's Hospital, on the following morning. I have since received several supplies from Mr. Bullock, and have used it in a variety of cases; but, before I describe the results of its application, it will be more convenient to give an account of its chemical constitution, and of those of its physical properties which are intimately connected with its physiological action.

It was discovered in 1795 by the associated Dutch chemists, Bondt, Deiman, Vantroostwyk, and Lauwerenburgh. It is formed by the combination of two volumes of chlorine and two of olefiant gases. The latter, representing one atom, contains four atoms of carbon and four of hydrogen, and is considered to be a hydruret of acetyle,— acetyle being a hypothetic base consisting of four carbon and three hydrogen. When the two atoms of chlorine combine with the hydruret of acetyle, the following is, since the investigations of Regnault, believed to be what takes place. One atom of chlorine displaces an atom of hydrogen, and the hydruret of acetyle is converted into chloride of acetyle, whilst the other atom of chlorine combines with the displaced hydrogen, forming hydrochloric acid, and the two products at the same time uniting, hydrochlorate of chloride of acetyle is the result; and this is the chemical name of Dutch liquid in recent authors. This body is curiously connected with the discovery of chloroform, as was pointed out by Dr. Pereira in a communication on the history of the latter medicine.* Dr. Thomas Thomson, in the edition of his Chemistry published in 1810, gave the name of chloric ether to Dutch liquid, and stated that a solution of it in spirit was useful in medicine as a diffusible stimulant. Some years after this, Mr. Guthrie, a chemist in America, obtained a liquid by the distillation of spirit and water with bleaching powder, which he considered to contain the chloric ether of Dr. Thomson dissolved in spirit; and this product,

which, in fact, consisted of chloroform and alcohol, was used for some time in medicine under the name of chloric ether. In 1831, Soubeiran found that this preparation did not contain Dutch liquid—the chloric ether of Dr. Thomson; and the following year Liebig also made an analysis of it; but, failing to discover the hydrogen in the chloroform, he considered that it was composed of chlorine and carbon; and after this time the medicine was often called ter-chloride or sesqui-chloride of carbon. There are various chlorides of carbon which have been discovered by Faraday and Regnault; but they are very difficult to make, and I believe that none of them have ever been on sale, either for medical or other purposes, and that the so-called chlorides of carbon which have been used in medicine were all of them solutions of chloroform, of which body Dumas was the first to ascertain the true nature and composition.

Dutch liquid is somewhat heavier than water, having a specific gravity of 1·247. It boils at 180° Fah. It is very sparingly soluble in water, and the specific gravity of its vapour is 3·4484. In sensible properties it very nearly resembles chloroform; and hence, probably, the reason of Mr. Guthrie, when he discovered the latter substance, mistaking it for Dutch liquid. The odour is not quite so fruit-like as that of chloroform, and the vapour feels less pungent; but the reason of this is that a smaller quantity of vapour is given off from Dutch liquid than from chloroform; for I find that when the two vapours are diluted to the same extent—for instance, till the air contain five per cent., and inhaled from a balloon, there is then no difference in the pungency. The physical properties of Dutch liquid which are most intimately connected with its narcotic action, when inhaled, are its volatility and solubility. From some experiments before related it was concluded that in the second degree of narcotism the blood contains one-fiftieth part as much as it would dissolve, and in the fourth degree one twenty-fifth part. These experiments have been repeated with the liquid quite free from impurity, and the results obtained were the same.

I have endeavoured to ascertain the solubility of Dutch liquid as accurately

---

* Med. Gaz. vol. xl. p. 953.

as possible, by admitting small quantities of water to air saturated with the vapour, and confined over mercury in a graduated receiver. The average of a number of experiments gives 1·7 volume of vapour as the quantity that one volume of water will dissolve ; and, the liquid being 321 times as heavy as its vapour at 100°, it results that, at this temperature, one part of the liquid would require 189 parts of water to dissolve it.

If the average quantity of serum in the body be assumed to be the same as in treating of chloroform, and a calculation be made of the kind there given,* it will be found that the amount of Dutch liquid in the blood, in the second degree of narcotism, is rather more than twenty minims, and in the fourth degree forty-one minims. In the third degree the amount would be intermediate, viz. about thirty minims. These quantities are nearly twice as large as in the case of chloroform ; and this agrees exactly with what I have met with in practice, since nearly twice as much Dutch liquid has been required to cause insensibility as would have been required of chloroform. To estimate the strength of this substance when inhaled, its volatility requires to be taken into account, in addition to the above data. Whilst 100 cubic inches of air at 60° will take up 14 cubic inches of chloroform, they will only take up seven cubic inches of Dutch liquid; and the vapour, moreover, is not so heavy as that of chloroform,—consequently it is not half so volatile. This makes the difference in strength between the two agents still greater. To exhibit more accurately their relative power, the quantity of air may be calculated that a patient would require to breathe, when saturated by either of the two vapours at 60°, in order to be rendered insensible. Eighteen minims is the average amount of chloroform in the blood in the third degree of narcotism, the stage usually required for a surgical operation, and as about as much is expired again without being absorbed, thirty-six minims is about the quantity inhaled before an operation. This would require only 257 cubic inches of air to take it up if saturated at 60°, the air becoming expanded to 294 cubic inches.

* Vol. xli. p. 850.

Thirty minims of Dutch liquid require to be absorbed, as stated above, to induce the same amount of insensibility, and sixty minims would have to be inhaled. This quantity requires 904 cubic inches of air to allow it to be converted into vapour at 60°, the air being expanded to 967 cubic inches, an amount more than three times as great as requires to be inhaled in the case of chloroform ; and consequently Dutch liquid has less than one-third the power of the former when inhaled in a similar way. Sulphuric ether is rather stronger than Dutch liquid— the quantity of air saturated with its vapour that is required to induce insensibility being rather more than 800 cubic inches.

For the reasons given above, Dutch liquid is much slower in its action than chloroform ;* and whilst the chief endeavour in giving chloroform is to prevent the air from getting too strongly charged with the vapour, in giving Dutch liquid the endeavour is to get the air to take up sufficient of it. In one case, indeed, that of an infant in King's College Hospital, on which Mr. Fergusson operated for nævus, it failed to induce insensibility with the inhaler I was using (one contrived for chloroform), although continued for three or four minutes, and rather than cause further delay chloroform was used.

For reasons similar to those which render Dutch liquid slower in its action, when its effects are once produced they are more persistent than those of chloroform. Medicines so volatile as these escape from the system almost exclusively by the lungs; and as the quantity of Dutch liquid in the blood during insensibility is greater than that of chloroform, it would be longer in escaping, even if it could be exhaled at the same rate ; but, being less volatile, it cannot. There is a continual tendency to equilibrium between the elastic force of the vapour in the blood and that in the air contained in the pulmonary cells : and if the blood contain, for instance, one-thirtieth part as much of a volatile liquid as it could

* A preparation consisting of equal parts of chloroform and spirit was fraudulently introduced into the drug-market last spring, and sold to a considerable extent as Dutch liquid, although not containing any of that body. This counterfeit liquid would cause insensibility with nearly the same rapidity as chloroform.

dissolve, each cubic inch of air which reaches the cells of the lungs is capable of taking up one-thirtieth part as much as would saturate it at 100°; but this quantity is twice as great in the case of chloroform as in that of Dutch liquid. The longer duration of the effects of the latter substance as compared with the former has been very marked in a number of experiments on animals, as well as in practice.

Although, as above stated, a greater quantity of Dutch liquid than of chloroform is required to induce insensibility in the first instance, yet in cases requiring the continued inhalation of the vapour there is but little difference in the amount used; since, from the more persistent effect of Dutch liquid, it does not require to be repeated so often.

The following are the cases in which I have tried the effects of Dutch liquid :—

1. On March 21, 1849, a young woman, about 25 years of age, inhaled it, in the out-patients' room of St. George's Hospital, previous to having a tooth drawn. She was nervous and hysterical, and was alarmed at the inhalation, although very anxious to avoid the pain. She inhaled from the apparatus described before,* between one and two minutes, when she strongly requested to leave off. The tooth, a first lower molar, firmly fixed, was immediately extracted with the forceps by Mr. Parkinson, dresser to the surgeon for the week. The patient cried out slightly as the tooth came out. She said afterwards that the removal of the tooth did not hurt her so much as the lancing of the gum on a previous occasion. In a few minutes the partial stupor caused by the vapour had subsided. This patient was not rendered quite unconscious, but the sensibility, and consequently the pain, were apparently diminished.

2. Another young woman inhaled the Dutch liquid immediately afterwards. She breathed it very steadily. The pulse became increased a little in frequency and force soon after she began to inhale, and the face at the same time became slightly flushed. There was no further symptom, and no alteration in her appearance till nearly four minutes had elapsed, when volun-

tary motion ceased in the eyes and eyelids, and the pupils were turned upwards. The inhalation was now discontinued when she had inhaled just four minutes. The muscles of the jaw were rather rigid, but the mouth was easily opened by making a little pressure on the chin, and a bicuspid tooth was extracted with the forceps by Mr. Parkinson, without causing the least flinch, cry, or altered expression of countenance on the part of the patient. Immediately after the tooth was extracted she opened her eyes, looking bewildered at first, but in one minute after the inhalation ceased she regained her usual expression, and began to wash out her mouth. She said that she had felt nothing. Three minutes afterwards she left the hospital feeling well. The narcotism, in this case, just reached the third degree, and there was complete immunity from pain, as indeed there generally is under the effects of chloroform carried to the same extent, when it is inhaled slowly. The recovery was as prompt as it usually is from chloroform; but it should be noticed that when the inhalation of that vapour is left off just when the symptoms reach the point indicated in the above case, the patient usually begins to recover immediately, even before there would be time to extract a tooth. Two fluid drachms of Dutch liquid had been put into the inhaler, and it was not quite all used by these two patients. A drachm more was added when the next patient commenced to inhale.

3. This patient was a labouring man, between 30 and 40 years of age. Soon after beginning to inhale he commenced to laugh, and he kept the corners of his mouth stretched so widely apart that it was difficult to make the face-piece fit exactly. In about five minutes he appeared to have lost his consciousness, and he muttered incoherently. He soon afterwards became unruly, and was with difficulty kept in the chair. The conjunctiva remained sensible, and he flinched when a hair of his face was pulled. Although he inhaled a few minutes longer, he did not become further affected; the reason of this being, as I afterwards found, that the Dutch liquid in the inhaler was finished. There was great difficulty in getting the mouth open, not from spasm but from voluntary resist-

* Vol. xlii. p. 843.

ance exerted under the influence of some obscure dream. The patient flinched as the tooth was extracted; but on recovering his consciousness two or three minutes afterwards, he said that he had felt nothing. The truth probably is, that the feeling had been obscure, and there was no recollection of it. He complained, however, of giddiness, and began to look pale and sick. In a few minutes he vomited, and then complained of headache. He was complaining of headache and sickness half an hour afterwards, when I left him, expecting that these symptoms would soon subside. But I afterwards found that they continued so severe, with occasional vomiting, that he was kept in the hospital till the following morning, when he left, but came back in the forenoon, complaining that he could not go on with his work. Mr. Hammerton ordered him some medicine containing ammonia, and directed him to return the next morning if he should not feel well. He did not apply again.

This is the only case in which I have seen Dutch liquid followed by distressing sickness or headache; and the result might have been the same if chloroform or ether had been used, as such symptoms do now and then follow their use, though rarely to the same extent as in this case.

4. In the above cases the water bath of the inhaler was at the temperature of 60°; in this case it was raised to 70°. Fifty minims of the medicine were put into the inhaler, and a little girl, six years old, inhaled for two minutes. At the end of this time she became insensible, the pupils of the eyes being turned upwards. A decayed molar tooth was extracted without causing the least flinch or cry. In about a minute after the inhalation ceased, the child became conscious, but staggered on attempting to walk. She vomited a little, two or three minutes after this, but in a few minutes more was free from sickness, and pretty well. The fifty minims were not all consumed by this patient.

5. The subject of this case was a patient of Mr. Marshall, of Greek Street, in labour with her second child, on April 24. I exhibited twenty minims of Dutch liquid (all I had with me at the time) during the last three or four pains which expelled the fœtus. The patient ceased to complain, but continued her expulsive efforts. She was not rendered quite unconscious, but her sufferings were greatly alleviated, being, as she said afterwards, much less severe than before, whilst without the inhalation they would have been much greater. Mr. Marshall was present and attending to the labour. In this and the next three cases the vapour was administered by means of a small inhaler, which I commonly use for giving chloroform in midwifery cases; it consists of the same face-piece which forms part of my other inhalers, and of a short curved metallic tube, lined with bibulous paper.

6. Having expressed a wish to Dr. Murphy, Professor of Midwifery in University College, to try Dutch liquid in some cases of labour, I was called on by him on the day on which the last of the above cases occurred, and accompanied him to a patient of Mr. Jakins, of Osnaburg Street, who had been forty-eight hours in this, which was her first labour. Dr. Murphy, who is about to give the particulars of this and the next case to the profession, found it necessary to divide a thick dense band, extending across the vagina, and also to make an artificial os uteri, and deliver with the forceps. Half a drachm of the liquid being inhaled, it gradually induced a state of unconsciousness, during which the speculum vaginæ was introduced; the uterine contractions and slight expulsive efforts continued as before. A little more Dutch liquid was put into the inhaler, from time to time, so as to keep the patient unconscious. The pupils of the eyes were turned upwards during part of the time. No mental excitement or muscular rigidity was occasioned. Dr. Murphy proceeded to make an artificial os uteri, and to divide the ligamentous band. These operations were partly performed when my stock of Dutch liquid, about three fluid drachms, was all used. It had kept up insensibility for about an hour. Chloroform was now given, so as to keep the patient constantly insensible to the end of the delivery. There was little appreciable alteration in the symptoms on passing from the use of one vapour to that of the other. The effects induced were of the same kind, but they were produced with much less inhalation in the case of chloroform;

a few inspirations, now and then, with the valve partly open, sufficed instead of the previous more lengthy inhalation, with the valve closed. The delivery was effected with the forceps about an hour after the inhalation of chloroform commenced, half a fluid ounce of which was used, being a larger quantity than was used of Dutch liquid in the same period; but the patient was kept more deeply insensible during the whole of this latter period than in some part of the first hour, when the operation had not yet commenced. The child was born alive, but breathed feebly, and died next day. The placenta was expelled without hæmorrhage a few minutes after the birth of the child. The patient was quite conscious ten or fifteen minutes after the inhalation was discontinued; and after being bandaged and placed in a comfortable posture, she fell asleep, and slept almost uninterruptedly for twelve hours. She recovered very favourably.

7. On May 18, I administered the Dutch liquid at the request of Dr. Murphy, to a primipara, 35 years of age, who had been 48 hours in labour, when he resolved to deliver with the forceps. Half a drachm was put into the inhaler : the patient objected to the vapour at first, on account of its pungency, but afterwards inhaled readily, and in about two minutes appeared unconscious, the pupils being turned upwards, and the eyelids firmly closed, and resisting the attempt to open them. Dr. Murphy now began to introduce the forceps, and the patient cried out a little : another half drachm of the liquid was put in, and she soon became quiet, and was kept insensible till the birth of the child, which was effected in less than half an hour. She talked in a rambling manner about some ordinary topic once or twice during the inhalation, and also a few minutes after it was discontinued. Two fluid drachms were used in all. The placenta was expelled ten minutes after the birth of the child; soon after this the patient vomited; and fifteen minutes after the birth (the time when the inhalation was left off), the patient began to regain her consciousness. She recovered very favourably, and the child is living.

8. The Dutch liquid was administered in a case of cholera that Mr. Marshall, of Greek Street, requested me to see with him. The patient was a child seven years old, which had been ill twelve hours. The stools were copious and watery, and devoid of fæcal colour or odour; the vomiting was constant and severe; the features were sunken, and the pulse was about 160 in the minute, and so feeble as to be felt with difficulty. There were jactitation and great uneasiness, the latter probably resulting from cramps. Twenty minims were inhaled, which produced a state of unconsciousness and quiet, from which the little girl awoke in ten minutes. The same quantity was again inhaled, with a like effect, and of rather longer duration. The pulse was improved by the inhalation, being rendered stronger and less frequent; but the chief symptoms of the disorder went on as before. The child recovered.

The relief from inhalation of chloroform in cholera has generally been greater than this in the cases I have witnessed, the unconsciousness having generally merged into a natural sleep, of from half an hour to two hours and a half in duration, during which time of course the patients were free both from sickness and spasm. Two of the cases were also under the care of Mr. Marshall. I attribute the different action in the above case to some difference in the state of the patient, rather than in the properties of the narcotic.

9. On July 18, a boy, nine years old, inhaled Dutch liquid in the out-patients' room of St. George's Hospital, from the balloon described in my last communication. Each hundred cubic inches of air in the balloon contained four minims of the liquid, or a small fraction over four cubic inches of the vapour. In two minutes consciousness was removed; he then began to resist the further inhalation, but with a little trouble was got to inhale two minutes longer. He was not narcotised beyond the second degree. Voluntary motion was never abolished, but the sensibility of the conjunctiva was diminished. Two incisor teeth of the first set were extracted without being felt (probably without the inhalation there would have been no great pain). He was laid on the bed, and in two minutes recovered his consciousness, but staggered on getting up. In about ten minutes the effects of the vapour had

apparently gone off. He inhaled about 1000 cubic inches, and consequently 40 minims of Dutch liquid; this quantity of chloroform would have rendered an adult of twice his weight fully as insensible as he was, if not more so.

The result of my observations and investigations is, that I cannot unite with Mr. Nunnelly in his general praises of Dutch liquid. The only advantages which it possesses over chloroform, in any case, are such as are connected with its slower action and more persistent effects, — properties that Mr. Nunnelly failed to recognize. In all other respects its effects appear to be the same as those of chloroform. It is undoubtedly a very safe anæsthetic; but I doubt very much whether practitioners would be content to wait for its slower action, after they have been accustomed to use chloroform, even if it could be obtained at the same cost, of which there is no prospect. In whatever way Dutch liquid might be used, it would not suddenly occasion a fatal accident without giving due warning; in this respect it resembles ether. Advantage might be taken of its more persistent effect in some operations in the face, in which it is difficult to administer a vapour after the surgeon commences; and also in cases in which the operator is without an assistant, and has to make his patient insensible first, and then to perform his operation. In obstetric practice it would perhaps be more convenient than chloroform, when only one medical man is present, as he might intrust the inhaler to the nurse, and look up two or three times in a minute to give directions; but when there is a practitioner entirely to superintend the inhalation, chloroform has the advantage, as it can be given to the requisite extent just as each pain commences, and the patient can be allowed to recover from its effects, more or less, between every pain.

————

PART XIII.

Action of Alcohol compared with that of Chloroform and Ether.

Experiments on frogs with alcohol—On fishes, with alcohol, chloroform, and ether—Quantity of alcohol necessary to cause drunkenness—To cause death.

Anæsthetic effects of alcohol—Liebig's views of the action of alcohol—their application to ether and chloroform—Objections to these views.

I FEEL that I ought to apologise to the readers of the MEDICAL GAZETTE for the great length of time that has been allowed to elapse before the completion of these papers. The delay has not arisen from any want of anxiety on my part to bring the subject to a conclusion, but from finding, as I proceeded with it, that it was desirable to repeat many experiments and institute fresh ones, the performance of which occupied a great deal of time.

In order to enter on the investigation of the *modus operandi* of ether and chloroform with every advantage, it is desirable to ascertain whether or not alcohol, which, in its chemical constitution and general physiological properties, considerably resembles these medicines, is identical with them in its action. It was previously stated* that alcohol, pyroxilic spirit, and acetone, which are miscible with water in all proportions, confirm the general rule then laid down, that the power of volatile narcotic substances of the class we are considering is in the inverse ratio of their solubility, as a large quantity of the above three liquids requires to be taken to produce narcotism. It afterwards occurred to me that experiments might be instituted to ascertain whether alcohol and the other two liquids obey exactly the law which we found to apply to chloroform, ether, and a number of other bodies. Experiments to determine this point could not easily be made on animals that breathe air exclusively, on account of the length of time that the vapour would continue to be absorbed; but, by employing frogs and fishes, the end could be attained. In the experiments previously related, it was found that the second degree of narcotism was caused when the serum of the blood contained about a fifty-sixth part as much of the chloroform, ether, or other substance examined, as it would hold in solution. Now, if the rule apply to alcohol, the second degree of narcotism ought to be induced when the amount of spirit is equal to one fifty-sixth of the volume of the serum.

The following are some of the expe-

* Vol. xlii. p. 333.

E

[65]

riments undertaken to determine this point.

Exp. 47.—A frog was placed in a shallow glass jar, capable of holding a pint. Seven ounces of water, mixed with a fluid drachm and a quarter of rectified spirit of wine, were put into the jar. The spirit consisted of 80 per cent. absolute alcohol, of which it consequently contained one drachm; and, as there are fifty-six drachms in seven ounces, the water contained one part of alcohol in fifty-six. It was the early part of March; and the frog, although quite sensible, was not very lively. When enclosed in the jar, it sat, with the head above the water, breathing the air at the rate of ninety respirations in the minute. As the jar was covered by a plate of glass, the air it contained would soon become charged with vapour of alcohol to the same relative extent as the water; that is to say, it would contain 1-56th part as much as if saturated at the same temperature, and the tendency of the absorption, by both the lungs and skin of the frog, would be to establish an equilibrium between the quantity of alcohol in the fluids of its body and that in the surrounding water, when the blood of the frog would consist of about 1-56th part spirits. Two hours after the commencement of the experiment, the strength of the frog appeared to be diminished, and it had a difficulty in keeping its nostrils above the water. It was breathing irregularly, and much less frequently than before. At the end of four hours its head was under the surface, and it was not breathing. Being taken out for a minute or two, it moved its head and limbs feebly, but apparently in a voluntary manner, but did not attempt to breathe. It was replaced in the jar, and left for the night, with its head beneath the surface, the jar being covered as before. The next morning, twelve and a half hours from the beginning of the experiment, the frog was found with its nostrils slightly raised above the surface of the spirit and water, and breathing gently and slowly. Being taken out, it was found to flinch slightly on the skin being pinched, and was able to crawl slowly, chiefly by the use of the anterior extremities. It recovered perfectly in the course of the day. The temperature of the room during this experiment was 50 Fahr.

Exp. 48. Another frog was placed in the same jar, with seven ounces of water, containing two and a half fluid drachms of the same spirit, the strength being consequently one part of alcohol in twenty-eight parts. In about an hour and a half the frog seemed feeble, and had difficulty in keeping its nostrils above the surface. At the end of two hours, its head had sunk beneath the surface, but the respiratory movements were going on, though feebly, and it seemed to be swallowing the liquid. At the end of three hours the lower jaw had fallen, and the mouth was open, but there were slight respiratory movements of the hyoid bones. There were feeble muscular twitches (subsultus tendinum) observed occasionally. A support was at this time placed under the anterior extremities of the frog, to keep its head above the surface of the water. It was found to be totally insensible to pinching. Its mouth continued open, and the feeble respiratory movements went on. At the end of five hours it was breathing very gently, and very slight twitchings of the toes could be observed occasionally. Seven hours and a quarter from the commencement of the experiment, the respiration had ceased. The frog was taken out, and showed no signs of life at first; but, on closely observing it, slight quivering movements of the toes, and of different parts of the muscles just beneath the skin, could be seen It was exposed to the air in a shallow dish containing a very little fresh water. In two hours after its removal, feeble respiratory movements could be occasionally observed. The breathing gradually became quite re-established, and seven hours after its removal it had recovered both sensibility and voluntary motion. The next day it seemed pretty well, and had resumed its colour, having been rendered nearly black whilst narcotised. The other frog also became much darker in colour, whilst under the influence of the spirit, in the previous experiment.

In the former of the above experiments the frog appeared to be in the second degree of narcotism, sensibility and voluntary power being impaired, but not abolished. In the last experiment the narcotism reached, and apparently rather exceeded, the fourth degree. The effect produced was nearly the same as that caused by one twenty-sixth part as much chloroform as the blood would dissolve, in one of the frogs, the subject of Experiment 15, formerly related; and rather more than the effect produced by one thirty-second part as much ether as the blood would dissolve, in a frog used in Exp. 28.

Exp. 49.—The frog employed in Exp. 47, being in good health, was, four days afterwards, placed in the same jar with nine ounces of water, containing five fluid drachms of rectified spirit of 80 per cent., equivalent to half an ounce of absolute alcohol; the proportion of alcohol being, consequently, one in eighteen of the mixture. At first the frog made some attempts to get out. At the end of seven minutes it withdrew its head voluntarily beneath the surface, and ceased to breathe; but two or three minutes afterwards it raised it again above the surface, and breathed the air. Twenty minutes from the commencement, it appeared to have a difficulty in keeping its nostrils above the surface, and now and then made an abortive attempt to leap up. The eyelids were half closed, and the cornea looked dim. At the end of half an hour it was lying on its belly without any sign of life. A support was placed under it to keep its head above the surface, and feeble respiratory movements recommenced. Three quarters of an hour from the beginning of the experiment, the respiration had entirely ceased, and no external sign of life remained. It was left an hour longer in the jar, and was taken out after being exposed to the spirit and water, and the vapour given off from it, for an hour and three quarters. No pulsation of the heart could be observed externally, but on removing a portion of the integuments and sternum with the scissors, the heart was found to be pulsating feebly. The frog was placed again in the spirit and water, being laid on its back, so that the heart could be observed. It was noticed to continue pulsating feebly for half an hour. Being left for two hours, it was found at the end of that time that the action of the heart had entirely ceased. As only one or two drops of blood were lost in exposing the heart, and as frogs at the temperature at which this experiment was performed (52° Fah.) can live almost altogether without the pulmonary respiration, it is probable that the action of the heart was arrested by the narcotic effect of the alcohol; and it was found in experiments 42 and 43, formerly related, that one eighteenth part as much

of the vapour of chloroform as the blood would dissolve, had the effect of arresting the action of the heart in frogs.

Exp. 50.—Two fluid drachms and a half of rectified spirit, equivalent to a quarter of a fluid ounce of absolute alcohol, were mixed with sufficient water to make up fourteen ounces, which, consequently, contained one part of alcohol in fifty-six parts. This was put into the glass jar before used, and a small gold fish, weighing two drachms and a half, was put in. The jar was covered, to prevent loss of spirit by evaporation. After a few minutes the fish seemed rather more active than before it was put in. At the end of twenty minutes it no longer regarded, or was frightened by, any object touching the jar, and it began to oscillate from side to side in swimming, and to incline to one side when still. Half an hour from the beginning of the experiment it was swimming very much on its side. It did not become appreciably more narcotised, although it remained in the water and spirit until two hours had expired. It struggled whilst being removed into fresh water. In half an hour after its removal it had partially recovered, and when next observed, two or three hours later, it was in its usual state.

Exp. 51.—Another small gold fish, weighing rather more than three drachms, was placed, in the same manner, in water containing one twenty-eighth part by measure of alcohol. In less than ten minutes the fish began to move about violently. Soon afterwards these movements became irregular and ill directed, the fish being unable to preserve the perpendicular position, and it no longer observed objects brought close to the jar. It continued, every now and then, to move about violently, and somewhat convulsively, till three quarters of an hour had expired, when it became quieter, floating on its side, and moving only occasionally. The opercula moved, but not regularly. At the end of an hour it had ceased to move its body and fins altogether, and a few minutes later it was found that the opercula did not move. It was placed in fresh water, and in a few minutes the opercula began to move, at first at long intervals, but in half an hour the respiration was regular, and the fish was beginning to move its body. The next morning it appeared quite well.

In Exp. 50 the fish was in the second degree of narcotism, and in the last experiment there was complete insensibility, and the fish would soon have died, probably not from absorption of additional spirit, but because the utmost extent of narcotism cannot be long continued without extinguishing the vital powers.

In some experiments with pyroxilic spirit, or wood naphtha, the same effects were produced on fishes, when it was mixed with water in the same proportion as the alcohol in the two last experiments; but the fishes died several hours afterwards, through the poisonous action of the naphtha, having first, in a great measure, recovered their sensibility and voluntary power.

The two following experiments are introduced for the purpose of showing that chloroform and ether act on fishes in the same way as on other animals.

Exp. 52. — Six fluid drachms of water in a small evaporating dish were placed on a plate of glass, by the side of a small dish containing chloroform; the two dishes were covered by a bell-glass, ground at the edge, to fit air-tight on the glass plate, and left till the next day, in order that the water might be saturated with chloroform, by absorbing it in the form of vapour. As soon as the bell-glass was removed, the small dish of water was put quickly into two pints of water, in which a gold fish was swimming, in a glass jar capable of holding three pints, and the jar was covered to prevent loss by evaporation. In ten minutes the fish began to oscillate a little in swimming. At the end of twenty minutes it was swimming frequently on its side, and then again recovering its balance. Half an hour from the beginning of the experiment the fish floated for a minute or two on its side, at the surface of the water, without moving its body or fins; then it began to swim about again for a time, and it continued occasionally to move for a short time, and then again to appear lethargic, until it was removed and put into fresh water, three hours after the commencement of the experiment. It struggled a little whilst being lifted out of the water. In an hour it had in a great measure recovered, and next day was as well as before. The water saturated with chloroform composed a fifty-fourth of the whole, which consequently contained one fifty-fourth part

as much chloroform as it would dissolve, and the fish was in the second degree of narcotism.

Exp. 53.—A fluid drachm of ether was mixed with two pints of water, and a gold fish put into it, and the jar was covered, as in the former experiment. As water is capable of dissolving one-tenth of its volume of ether, the water in this experiment contained one thirty-second part as much as it would dissolve. The fish was but little affected during the first hour, but at the end of an hour and a half it inclined to one side in swimming. When two hours had elapsed it was floating completely on its side, and had ceased to move its fins. It was taken out and put into fresh water. It moved a little on being handled. In about ten minutes it began to swim, and the effects of the ether gradually and completely went off.

As the deeper degrees of narcotism cannot be long continued without dangerously depressing the vital actions, so, with an agent whose effects last so long as those of alcohol, a state of complete coma cannot be induced at all without risk, especially if the body be exposed to a low temperature. Ordinary drunkenness does not exceed the second degree of narcotism; the popular term of dead drunk being often applied to a state of sleep from which the individual is still capable of being roused to a state of incoherent consciousness. In order to estimate the quantity of spirit that would be required to induce the second degree of narcotism in a man having the average amount of blood, 410 fluid ounces, which were taken as the amount of serum in the body in the earlier parts of this article, may be divided by 56, which will give seven ounces one drachm, a quantity of alcohol equal to rather more than fifteen ounces, or three-quarters of a pint of proof spirit. This is a quantity which, I believe, agrees pretty well with general experience. Less than twice this amount, if taken all at once, and on an empty stomach, so as to be quickly absorbed, ought, according to the above considerations, to prove fatal; and there have been many instances of such a result.

A few years ago a man drank a bottle of gin, in the Haymarket, for a wager. He was soon in a state of profound insensibility, and the late Mr.

Read, the instrument maker, informed me that when he applied the stomach-pump at the police station, in the presence of a medical gentleman, the stomach was found to be quite empty. The man shortly afterwards died. The quantity of absolute alcohol in a bottle (twenty-four ounces) of strong gin is about thirteen ounces. In the fifth case in Dr. Ogston's paper on intoxication,* a woman lost her life by drinking less than a bottle of whiskey; and I believe that it is only by dividing the dose, and thus distributing its effect over a longer time, that any person can, with impunity, take a quantity of spirit exceeding this. The two bottles of wine which, when drinking was less unfashionable than at present, some persons could take after dinner, without being rendered altogether incapable, would contain, according to Mr. Brande's table, from nine to twelve ounces of alcohol; but this quantity was consumed during a protracted sitting, and after eating food, which would further retard its absorption. The difference in susceptibility to the influence of alcohol, though existing to some extent, is not so great as it appears to be. The real difference is more in the way in which the mind is affected by it. A person who is excited evinces the effects of a moderate quantity, which are not so apparent on one who is not excited; whilst to make both individuals quite insensible, the quantity, as in the case of ether or chloroform, would probably not differ more than the size of the individuals, or rather the quantity of blood they might contain. With respect to the large amount of wine and spirits that patients in a state of extreme debility sometimes take without being apparently intoxicated, the following remarks may be made. Such persons are usually incapable of showing excitement under the influence of narcotics; and, as the alcohol is given in divided doses, which are insufficient to cause insensibility or coma, the effects which are really produced pass unnoticed. Long habit has some effect in enabling a person to take a larger quantity of alcoholic liquor: this, however, does not arise altogether from the diminished action of the spirit, but partly from experience of the muddled condition, which enables him to control

his actions to some extent, and to go about his affairs with a sort of sober aspect when very unfit for business. The woman whose case is quoted above, and who was killed by less than a bottle of whiskey, was a drunkard; and, at all events, the habit of drinking alcohol has no power of enabling persons to increase the dose in the extraordinary manner in which that of opium can be increased.

The amount of anæsthesia from alcohol is apparently as great, in proportion to the narcotism of the nervous centres attending it, as from chloroform and ether. A case occurred in King's College Hospital illustrating this. On Thursday night, the 21st of December, 1848, Mr. Fergusson performed amputation of the leg on an elderly man who had just before sustained a bad compound fracture. The man was very drunk, and Mr. Fergusson informed me that he evinced but little feeling, and did not seem aware of what was being done. He called out once during the operation that he had the cramp in his leg. When I questioned the patient a day or two afterwards, he said that he did not remember anything of the operation, and he supposed that chloroform had been administered to him. This, however, was not the case. Alcohol does not yield sufficient vapour, at ordinary temperatures, to cause insensibility by inhalation in a reasonable time; but, if no better means had been discovered, there can be no doubt that it would have been both practicable and allowable to prevent the pain of severe operations by getting the patient to swallow a large quantity of spirit and water. The end would have justified the means, and, in fact, rendered it as praiseworthy as it is disgraceful when resorted to for the purpose of supposed enjoyment, or to satisfy a craving which has resulted from a pernicious habit.

The general tendency of physiological researches had for some time been to prove that all the strictly animal functions resulted from the combination of the oxygen of the air with the constituents of the body, when Liebig* stated the position more fully and clearly than, as I believe, had previously been done. His attempted explanation of the physiological action of alcohol, which many persons were inclined to extend to that

---

* Edin. Med. and Sur. Jour. vol. xl.

* Animal Chemistry.

of ether, on its introduction for inhalation, is in accordance with these views, and is to the following effect*:—That, according to all the observations hitherto made, neither the expired air, nor the perspiration, nor the urine, contains any trace of alcohol after indulgence in spirituous liquors†; that the elements of alcohol combine with oxygen in the body, and that its carbon and hydrogen are given off as carbonic acid and water; that the elements of alcohol appropriate the oxygen of the arterial blood, which would otherwise have combined with the matter of the tissues, or with that formed by the metamorphosis of the tissues: and that thus the change of the tissues, and the muscular and other forces which would result from that change, are diminished. Whilst it may be admitted that alcohol diminishes the change of tissues and the functions connected with these changes, and will, indeed, be shown further on that this is true with regard also to the narcotic vapours treated of in this article, it can readily be proved that it is not by appropriating the oxygen in the blood that this diminution or suspension of the molecular change of tissues is effected. The following, amongst other considerations, show this :—First, the carbon and hydrogen of fat, starch, sugar, and gum, as Baron Liebig had the merit of showing, combine with oxygen in the blood, and are given off as carbonic acid gas and water; yet these substances are in no degree narcotic. Second, the carbon and hydrogen of chloroform, which in the laws of its action is almost, if not quite, identical with alcohol, could not possibly combine with oxygen sufficient to act in the way supposed. The amount of carbon and hydrogen in twenty-four minims of chloroform—the quantity which, as it was estimated on a previous occasion, exists in the blood of the adult in complete insensibility,—is only about four grains: an amount totally insignificant when compared to the oxygen which is continually absorbed in the lungs. And, third, if alcohol and the agents allied to it acted by appropriating the oxygen in the arterial blood, breathing air richer than usual in oxygen ought to prevent or arrest their narcotic action. But such is not the case: breathing even pure oxygen does not remove intoxication, or prevent

or remove the effects of narcotic vapours. The latter point I have ascertained as regards both the human subject and inferior animals, and have seen insensibility kept up in an animal by the ordinary amount of ether vapour, whilst its skin was of a bright vermilion colour, from the excess of oxygen in the blood.

PART XIV.

Chloroform passes off unchanged from the blood, in the expired air—Its detection in the urine—in the dead body—in an amputated limb—Remarks on the process for its detection.

At the end of the last paper, reasons were given for concluding that the effects of narcotic vapours were not due, as some had supposed, to the hydrogen and carbon they contain, combining with the oxygen of the air dissolved in the blood; and evidence was adduced to show that if such combination do take place, this would not explain their narcotic action. It still remained desirable to determine by experiment, if possible, whether these bodies are decomposed in the system, or pass off unchanged in the breath, or in other ways. With this view the following experiment was performed :—

Exp. 54.—Ten minims of chloroform were put into a hydrogen balloon, holding 300 cubic inches. The balloon was filled up with air, which I breathed backwards and forwards, in the way in which nitrous oxide gas is taken, for probably about two minutes. The word probably is used, because, after observing the watch for a minute and a half, I lost the recollection of what I was doing, and on recovering so as to observe the watch again, I found that another minute had elapsed, and that I had carefully lain aside the balloon in the meantime. Half a minute after this, and three minutes after beginning to inhale, I commenced to pass the expired air through a tube of hard glass, which was placed in readiness in a charcoal fire. To the further end of the tube were fitted other tubes connecting it with two Woolfe's bottles, each containing a solution of nitrate of silver. The respired air was taken in by the nostrils and breathed out by the mouth, passing first through the red hot tube, and afterwards through the solutions of nitrate of silver. This process was continued for four minutes.

---

* Ibid. p. 239.
† This we shall afterwards find to be incorrect.

The solution was rendered turbid, more especially that in the first bottle; being at first white, but shortly afterwards of a dark violet colour. At the end of twenty-five minutes from the inhalation, and when scarcely any appreciable effect of the chloroform remained on the feelings, I again breathed the expired air through the red-hot tube, the Woolfe's bottles having been removed, and a small tube moistened inside with solution of nitrate of silver having been attached. A slight precipitate of chloride of silver immediately appeared in the tube. The precipitate in the Woolfe's bottles having been washed and dried on the filter, was found to weigh 1·2 grain.

I have on other occasions, after inhaling chloroform, made the expired air to pass at once through a solution of nitrate of silver without the intervention of the red-hot tube, when not the least precipitate was occasioned; consequently, the chlorine which combined with the silver in the above experiment was the result of the decomposition of chloroform in the hot tube, and not in the circulation. As upwards of half a minute was allowed to elapse, during which several inspirations were taken between the conclusion of the inhalation and commencing to breathe through the tube, the lungs must have been completely emptied of the air taken from the balloon, and the vapour of chloroform must consequently have been exhaled from the blood. The further part of the experiment, performed twenty minutes later, more strongly proves this, and also shows that chloroform continues to be exhaled as long as any appreciable effects of it remain.

If all the chlorine of the chloroform united with the silver, the quantity of chloride obtained in four minutes, in the above experiment—viz. 1·2 grain, would indicate only 0·476 grain of chloroform. But I have found that on passing the vapour of a known quantity of chloroform through a red-hot tube, only about one-third of the chlorine is liberated, chiefly in the form of hydrochloric acid gas, and combines with the silver, as will be more fully explained further on: consequently, the above quantity of chloride of silver may be taken to indicate 1·428, or nearly a grain and a half of chloroform. It would not be easy to continue to test

for the whole of the vapour exhaled by the breath. Indeed, breathing through the tubes and liquids for four minutes, in the above experiment, was attended with some inconvenience. But when it is considered that part of the chloroform used must have remained in the balloon, that a further part must have been exhaled before beginning to breathe through the red-hot tube, and that the vapour was still being exhaled twenty-five minutes after the inhalation, the experiment must help to confirm the view that by far the greater part of the chloroform inhaled is exhaled again by the breath.

It is probable that a small portion of chloroform passes out by other channels than that of the expired air: the latter, however, offers such a ready and expeditious outlet, that the quantity excreted in any other way is, most likely, very minute. I have on four occasions examined urine passed after the inhalation of chloroform, by boiling it in a flask, and passing the vapour, first through a red-hot tube, and afterwards through a tube moistened inside with solution of nitrate of silver, and I only on one occasion obtained a very slight precipitate of chloride of silver.

The presence of chloroform can be detected in portions of the body removed by the surgeon, when the patient is under its influence, and in the bodies of animals killed by it. And as this part of the subject is interesting in a medico-legal as well as in a physiological point of view, I shall enter a little more minutely into the account of it than I might otherwise have done. In the Journal de Chemie Médicale for March, 1849, a process for the detection of chloroform in the blood is described in the following terms:—" In order to recognise the presence of chloroform in the blood, we take advantage of the property which this body possesses of being decomposed at a red heat, in giving rise to chlorine and hydrochloric acid. In order to perform the operation, it is sufficient to boil an ounce of blood for some time in a glass flask over the water bath. The vapour must pass through a tube heated to redness at one part, and of which the extremity is smeared interiorly with a mixture of iodide of potassium and paste of starch. A strip of paper moistened with the same mixture may also be put into the tube. If any chlorine be produced by the decomposition of chloroform, the strip of paper will be turned blue. In this way one part of chloroform in 10,000 of blood may be discovered." It is not stated in this article whether the chloroform detected had entered the blood during life, or had been added after its removal, though the former was probably meant

In employing this process I substituted solution of nitrate of silver for the starch and iodine test, considering that to obtain some of the chlorine as chloride of silver would be more satisfactory, in a medico-legal point of view, than merely showing the presence of something which decomposes the iodide of potassium. I find, also, that the nitrate of silver possesses other decided advantages. In the first place, it is a much more certain and delicate test. The iodine test is not acted on by hydrochloric acid, but only by the free chlorine, very little of which is produced by passing the vapour of chloroform through a red-hot tube, and that not constantly. Again, if there be a trace of chlorine to set free a little of the iodine, a little warm vapour, which is very apt to rush through the tube, whilst it does not affect the chloride of silver, may either prevent the blue colour of iodide of starch being developed, or suddenly discharge it, as I have seen. And lastly, the nitrate of silver test allows of a quantitative analysis being made, whilst the other does not admit of it. Dr. Alfred Taylor has, however, suggested to me to combine the two tests with a third one, by introducing a slip of starch paper moistened with solution of iodide of potassium, and also a slip of blue litmus paper, into another part of the tube, where it is not wet with the nitrate of silver. Used in this way, these additional tests may tend to confirm the evidence, and to meet objections that might possibly be made to the nitrate of silver test when used alone.

Before relating the experiments in which the presence of chloroform was detected in the body, it will be preferable to give some account of the decomposition which takes place when the vapour of that substance is passed through a red-hot tube. Soubeiran, when treating, in 1831,[*] of the body afterwards named chloroform, said, that

on passing it, in the form of vapour, through a tube of porcelain filled with small fragments of porcelain, and made red-hot, that a good deal of charcoal is deposited, and that a gas is produced formed almost entirely of hydrochloric acid; and that there is found besides a very small quantity of chlorine and of an inflammable gas. He added, that, unless the pieces of porcelain are so arranged in the tube as to delay the passage of the vapour, without obstructing it too much, there is more chlorine liberated, and a substance left in the tube which stains paper like an oil. Liebig[*] says of chloroform, "when its vapour is passed through a red-hot tube it is decomposed into carbon, hydrochloric acid, and a crystalline body which appears in long white needles." On another occasion[†] he says that this crystalline body is probably the perchloride of carbon discovered by Mr. Faraday.

I performed the following experiments with a view more particularly to ascertain whether any appreciable quantity of free chlorine is produced during the decomposition of chloroform at a red heat:—

a. Ten grains of chloroform were put into a dry retort, made out of a small green glass tube, and capable of holding only a drachm. The retort was heated gradually in the water bath. Its beak was kept red-hot by the flame of a spirit lamp, and communicated with two Woolfe's bottles, containing solution of nitrate of silver. Charcoal was deposited in the beak of the retort at the part where it was red-hot: half an inch from this part, on each side, there was a copious deposit of long, white, needle-shaped crystals, and, after a time, a reddish-brown oily-looking liquid appeared. The precipitate of chloride of silver, which was found almost exclusively in the first bottle, weighed, after being washed and thoroughly dried, 12·5 grains.

b. Ten grains of chloroform were put into a similar retort and treated in the same way, except that the beak of the retort opened under a receiver in the mercurial trough. The deposits in the tube of the retort were the same as before, and 9.15 cubic inches of gaseous matter were obtained in the receiver.

---

* Annales de Chimie et de Physique, t. xlviii. p. 135.

* Turner's Chemistry, 8th edit. p. 1009.
† Annales de Chimie, t. xlix.

The tenth of a cubic inch of water being passed through the mercury, 8·5 cubic inches of the gas were absorbed by it. Solution of potash absorbed one-tenth of a cubic inch more, and the remainder consisted almost, or entirely, of air expelled from the retort.

c. Ten grains of chloroform were treated in the same way as before, the beak of the small retort communicating with two Woolfe's bottles, the first of which contained only thirty minims of distilled water, and the second some solution of nitrate of silver. A very slight cloudiness was merely produced in this solution in the second bottle. The water in the first bottle being added, at the end of the process, to a solution of nitrate of silver, and the precipitate occasioned being boiled in nitric acid, washed, and thoroughly dried, was found to weigh 11·45 grains.

If one of the three atoms of chlorine which were contained in the chloroform were to combine with the single atom of hydrogen, the hydrochloric acid thus produced from ten grains would weigh 3·04 grains, and would suffice to form 12·08 grains of chloride of silver. In experiment a, the chloride of silver obtained exceeded this by a very little. In experiment b, any chlorine which might be developed would be absorbed by the mercury, and the 8·5 cubic inches of gas absorbed by the small quantity of water must have consisted of hydrochloric acid. The weight of it would be 3·24 grains—a very little more than ought by theory to result from the combination of one of the atoms of chlorine with the hydrogen of the formyle; and it would combine to form 12·7 grains of chloride of silver. In experiment c, the thirty minims of water, whilst they absorbed the hydrochloric acid gas, could absorb but a very minute quantity of chlorine, certainly less than the tenth of a grain, and consequently if a greater amount of chlorine than this had been evolved it must have passed on to the second bottle, and there caused a precipitate of chloride of silver. On precipitating with nitrate of silver, it will be observed that the quantity of chloride obtained was very nearly that which ought to be formed by the hydrochloric acid produced as suggested above. These experiments, then, tend to show, that if chlorine be produced by passing the vapour of chloroform through a red-hot tube, it must be in extremely small

quantity, and that consequently the proper tests to employ are those which indicate the presence of hydrochloric acid.

The following is a brief account of the experiments for the detection of chloroform in the body :—

Exp. 55.—Two kittens about a fortnight old were placed in a glass jar holding 120 cubic inches. Twelve minims of chloroform were dropped on a piece of blotting paper in the jar, and it was closed. In two minutes the kittens were both insensible, and in two minutes more one of them had ceased to breathe; the other continued to breathe feebly and irregularly for six minutes longer. On the following day one of the kittens was opened : there was no odour of chloroform perceptible in this, any more than in the numerous other animals that I have killed with it.

a. The lungs, liver, and kidneys of this kitten were placed in a wide-mouthed glass flask with two or three drachms of water. The flask was placed in the water bath, to which (common salt not being at hand) was added a little chloride of calcium, to increase the temperature somewhat. A tube passing through the cork of the flask was connected with one of hard glass, which was kept red-hot in the flame of a spirit lamp, and to the end of the latter tube was attached one wetted inside with solution of nitrate of silver. About the time that the contents of the flask began to boil, a white curdy precipitate appeared in the latter tube. This precipitate was rendered dark-coloured by the light. It was insoluble in nitric acid, and very soluble in ammonia.

b. Two days after the death of the kittens, the lungs, heart, liver, and kidneys of the other animal were treated in a similar manner. Soon after the water in the flask began to boil, a precipitate of chloride of silver appeared in the tube.

c. Three days after their death, the brains of both kittens were put into a flask without any water, and heated in the chloride of calcium bath, as the other parts had been. On this occasion the tube moistened with solution of nitrate of silver ended in a Woolfe's bottle containing a few minims of the same solution. By the time that the liquid which had exuded from the brains began to boil, a precipitate began to appear in the tube, and in a short time there was one also, to a slight extent, in the bottle.

F

The brains were kept boiling in their own serosity for an hour. On the following day heat was again applied to the flask containing the brains which had not been removed; the tube and Woolfe's bottle having, however, been cleaned and supplied with a fresh solution of nitrate of silver. Not the slightest precipitate was obtained on this occasion, although the brains were kept boiling for two hours.

d. Five days after its death one of the kittens was skinned, and the flesh of the limbs, together with the greater part of that of the body and neck, was stripped off and put into the flask and treated as before, with the exception that, instead of the solution of nitrate of silver, a slip of paper moistened with a mixture of starch and solution of iodide of potassium was placed in the farther end of the tube. After the flesh had been made to boil for a little time in its own juice, a small part of the paper was turned blue.

e. Six days after its death the skin of the other kitten was removed, and its flesh put into a flask and treated as above; on this occasion, solution of nitrate of silver being used as the test. The serosity of the flesh had scarcely began to boil, when a precipitate of chloride of silver began to appear, and was soon as copious as on any previous occasion, both in the tube and Woolfe's bottle. At this time the intestines of the kittens were beginning to be offensive, although the flesh used in the experiment was not at all decomposed. The bodies had lain on a table since the time of death, at the beginning of last May, when the temperature was cool. From the size of the animals, the quantity of chloroform inhaled by each was considerably less than a grain.

To try the delicacy of the above process, a grain of chloroform was dissolved in a hundred drops of rectified spirit, and one drop of this solution was dropped into a flask containing a thousand grains of water. On treating this as above described, a distinct precipitate of chloride of silver was obtained in the tube, thus indicating the presence of the hundredth part of a grain of chloroform in a thousand grains of water.

Exp. 56.—On May 9, some portions of muscle, nearly sufficient to fill a three-ounce bottle, were taken from the calf of the leg of a little boy, about five years old, which had just been amputated by Mr. P. Hewett, under the influence of chloroform, in St. George's Hospital. About four hours afterwards the pieces of muscle were put into a flask, and treated as before described, solution of nitrate of silver being the test applied. When the liquid exuding from the muscle had been boiling for about ten minutes the precipitate began to appear, and was soon very distinct.

On July 2d, I assisted Dr. Taylor, in the Laboratory of Guy's Hospital, in applying this process to a little of the blood of a man whose death had been occasioned by chloroform, six days previously. The blood, which had been kept in a stoppered bottle, measured six and a half drachms, was of a dark red colour, fluid, but rather thick, and did not smell offensive. It was put into a clean Florence oil flask, from which a tube proceeded which was made red-hot, and a further tube moistened inside with solution of nitrate of silver. The flask was heated in the water bath, to which, after a time, common salt was added. The process was continued for twenty minutes or more, and although a slight cloudiness was observed in the tube, no distinct precipitate of chloride of silver was obtained. It should be remarked that this small quantity of blood must necessarily have been exposed to the air, before it was put into the bottle, by which means it would lose a part of its chloroform.

At the suggestion of Dr. Taylor, some chloroform (about 8 drops) was put into a flask with an ounce of water, and in the further tube were placed, first, a slip of starch paper moistened with solution of iodide of potassium; next, a slip of blue litmus paper, and the distal extremity of the tube was wetted inside with solution of nitrate of silver. The intermediate tube being made red-hot, as soon as heat was applied to the water bath, the two pieces of paper and the solution of nitrate of silver began to be affected, almost simultaneously: the starch paper being rapidly rendered very blue, the change of colour beginning at one end and travelling rapidly along it.

On the same occasion, in order to try the delicacy of these tests, a drop of chloroform, which is equal to the third of a grain, was agitated in a minim measure with fifty minims of alcohol. Five minims of this solution were added to an ounce of water in a flask, which would consequently contain the thirtieth part of a grain of chloroform. A fresh tube being attached, containing the three tests before employed, and the flask being heated in the water bath, a decided effect was, in a little time, produced on all the tests. The starch paper was rendered blue; the litmus was turned red; and a very distinct precipitate was obtained in the solution of nitrate of silver.

EXP. 57.—July 13: Half a drachm of chloroform was diffused through a jar holding 670 cubic inches, and a kitten, weighing a little over thirteen ounces, was put in. In two minutes it was quite insensible, and at the end of ten minutes it died. On the 15th the kitten was opened, and the viscera of the chest, the liver, and the brain, weighing together nearly two ounces, were put into a flask and heated in the salt water bath. A tube coming from the flask was kept red-hot, and a further tube contained a slip of starch and iodide of potassium paper, and a slip of blue litmus, and terminated near the bottom of a Woolfe's bottle containing a few minims of solution of nitrate of silver. At the early part of the process, the edge of the starch paper seemed to be slightly changing colour, but after a little time no change of colour could again be observed in it. The blue litmus was very soon reddened, and the solution of nitrate of silver began to be turbid, and the turbidity increased for some time. The viscera were kept boiling in their serosity for half an hour.

On the following day other six ounces of the same kitten were put into the same flask; the intestines, skin, and larger bones being only left. Fresh starch paper was put into the tube which terminated in the bottle containing the same solution of nitrate of silver. After a little time the starch paper was decidedly darkened, at the corner nearest the flask, but only to a limited extent, which did not increase. The parts were kept boiling in their serosity for two hours, when the process was ended by the breaking of the tube at the part where it was red-hot, owing to a little condensed steam being projected against it. At the same moment the limited blueness of the starch paper was discharged. The tube being left lying on the table, it was found next day that the starch paper was very blue throughout its entire extent, from what cause I do not know. The precipitate of chloride of silver was separated by filtration, and but for an accident would have been dried and weighed. There appeared to be not less than the twentieth part of a grain of it.

There is no deposit of carbon in the red-hot part of the tube in this process, as the apparatus always contains sufficient air for the formation of the carbon into carbonic acid. The white needle-formed crystals previously mentioned are deposited, but not in sufficient quantity to be of service as a test. It is desirable to make the tubes proceeding from the flask incline a little upwards, so that the vapour which is condensed before reaching the red-hot part may flow back again. I consider that the solid organs of the body should be taken for analysis, in preference to the blood in a separate state, as that contained in the minute vessels is protected from the action of the air. The parts should be cut in pieces, and put into the flask, without any addition. The stomach should not be selected for examination by the above process, as the gastric juice contains a minute quantity of free hydrochloric acid, and hence the evidence would be liable to objection. The intestines also do not seem suitable parts for examination, as the sulphuretted hydrogen they might contain would interfere, more or less, with the tests. In other respects it matters little what part of the body be used, further than that the most vascular parts are the best. As regards a quantitative analysis, it results from some of the experiments, detailed in an early part of these papers,* that, in a case of death from chloroform, a quarter of a pound of any organ of average vascularity would contain about the twelfth part of a grain, which, if the whole of it were separated and decomposed, would produce about the tenth of a grain of chloride of silver.

The process above described does not prove the presence of chloroform itself, but only that of a volatile compound containing chlorine. In this respect it resembles the processes for the detection of arsenious acid and corrosive sublimate in the tissues, which prove only the presence of a compound of arsenic, or of mercury. The only compounds containing chlorine which are volatile at

---

* MED. GAZ., vol. xlii. p. 415.

the heat of boiling water, are substances such as chloride of ethyle, Dutch liquid, and some others, which resemble chloroform in their effects, but are none of them in common use. In order to be quite certain that the precipitate is no other salt of silver than the chloride, besides the tests of ammonia and nitric acid, solution of potash might be added to another portion of it, as recommended by Dr. Taylor, in treating of hydrochloric acid.* Potash does not change the chloride of silver without heat.

With these limitations and precautions the process is, I believe, liable to no fallacy. There are chlorides in the body, but they cannot be decomposed, except at a high temperature, and not till the part under examination should become dry, which, in the method here described, could not take place in the most protracted examination. Besides, I have made several examinations of parts not containing chloroform without meeting with anything that produced the slightest effect on the nitrate of silver, or on the starch or litmus test. The bodies of two kittens killed with the vapour of ether were submitted to the process, by portions at a time, which were made to boil in their own serosity for an hour or two, but not the least effect was produced on any of these tests. Hearing, in the beginning of May last, that chloroform was suspected, by some of the coroner's jury, to have been used in the case of a woman who was found dead, under mysterious circumstances, in the Wandsworth Road, I applied to Mr. John Parrott, who was polite enough to send me some portions of the body, including part of the brain and liver. They had been kept in a covered jar from the time they were removed from the body. The chemical examination commenced four days after death, whilst the parts were fresh, and although very carefully conducted, not the least effect was produced, either on the nitrate of silver or starch and iodine test.

---

* Medical Jurisprudence, p. 91.

PART XV.

Detection of ether in the expired air after inhalation—Detection of alcohol in the expired air after it had been taken into the stomach—The effects of chloroform and ether prolonged by causing the exhaled vapour to be re-inspired.

IN my last communication it was shown that the vapour of chloroform can be detected by chemical tests, as it exhales from the blood in the expired air. The strong odour of ether, which continues to be perceived for hours in the breath of persons who have inhaled it, is a pretty good indication that this medicine is exhaled from the blood in a similar manner. I thought it desirable, however, to have a more material proof of the fact, than that afforded by the odour, and therefore contrived and performed the following experiments:—

Exp. 58.—As a preliminary measure I passed the expired air for twenty minutes through strong sulphuric acid, inspiring by the nostrils, and expiring by the mouth, through a spiral tube immersed in cold water; a continuation of this tube afterwards dipping into half an ounce of sulphuric acid contained in a bottle. The acid was afterwards boiled in a small retort, the beak of which communicated with a gas receiver under water. No gas was obtained beyond the air expelled from the retort by the heat, and the acid was not changed in colour.

Exp. 59.—On the following day—August 1st, I inhaled three fluid drachms of ether gradually, in the course of four minutes, and was rendered almost unconscious. After waiting for a minute, in order that the lungs might be entirely emptied of the vapour remaining at the conclusion of the inhalation, I commenced to pass the expired air through sulphuric acid, the air first passing through a spiral tube immersed in iced water, to condense the watery vapour, as in the last experiment. This process was continued for twenty minutes. A few hours afterwards the sulphuric acid was placed in a small retort, the beak of which communicated with a receiver under water, and was heated with the flame of a spirit lamp. It was gradually rendered quite black by the heat, and 11·3 cubic inches of gas were obtained in the jar. The jar being transferred to the mercurial trough, and solution of caustic potash being introduced, the contents, after standing for an hour or two, and being agitated occasionally, till no further reduction of bulk would take place, were diminished to 3·9 cubic inches, showing an absorption of 7·4 cubic inches of carbonic acid gas. The jar being reversed, and a lighted taper being applied to its mouth, its remaining contents took fire, and burnt with a bluish flame. As 2·6 cubic inches of air were contained in the retort at the commencement of the process, the quantity of inflammable gas was probably 1·3 cubic inch.

Exp. 60.—On August 2nd, I again inhaled three fluid drachms of ether, and proceeded exactly as in the last experiment. The sulphuric acid was rendered black as before, and 7·6 cubic inches of gas were collected in the receiver. Potash absorbed 3·2 cubic inches of this, and the jar being reversed, and a lighted taper applied to its mouth, the remaining contents burnt with a flame which gradually descended in the jar to the surface of the mercury. Allowing for the air expelled from the retort, the quantity of combustible gas was 1·6 cubic inch.

Exp. 61.—In order to ascertain the nature of the inflammable gas produced, another experiment was performed, on a subsequent day. The same quantity of ether was inhaled, and the expired air was passed through sulphuric acid in the same manner. The acid was boiled in the retort, until 7·1 cubic inches of gas were obtained in the receiver, when the process was stopped. Solution of potassa being agitated in the gas absorbed 3·5 cubic inches. Two cubic inches of oxygen gas were added to the remaining 3·6 cubic inches, and a portion of the mixed gases was transferred to Dr. Ure's eudiometer. As it did not explode with the spark from a small electric machine, a small quantity of pure hydrogen gas was added, when explosion took place with the following result. The quantities are in hundredths of a cubic inch:—

Hydrogen	3·0
Oxygen, &c.	21·0
Total	24·0
After explosion	16·5
Loss of volume	7·5

being a diminution of three parts more than the hydrogen would occasion. The remaining 16·5 parts were agitated with a little solution of potassa, when a further diminution of about six parts took place; a little more than ten parts being left. This result shows that the inflammable gas under examination was carbonic oxide, which, in becoming converted into an equal volume of carbonic acid, consumes half its own volume of oxygen. The beak and upper part of the small retort contained 1·9 cubic inch of air, which would be necessarily expelled into the gas receiver, and when this and the oxygen afterwards added are subtracted, the remainder is in the same proportion, very nearly, as the carbonic acid produced by the explosion; consequently the gases obtained by heating the sulphuric acid were carbonic acid gas, and carbonic oxide.

In these experiments, the ether passing off in the expired air is in part absorbed by the sulphuric acid, and on the application of heat is decomposed into various products; the above gases being given off, and free carbon remaining in the acid, and rendering it black. Sulphurous acid gas is evolved, but is absorbed by the water. On adding a few minims of ether to half an ounce of sulphuric acid, and operating in the same way as in the above experiments, the same products were obtained. Alcohol, when heated with a large excess of sulphuric acid, yields the same products as ether; but as I had taken no kind of fermented liquor before inhaling the ether in the above experiments, these products must have resulted from the sulphuric ether.

From the general resemblance between the action of alcohol, ether, and chloroform, and from these substances being governed in their action by some of the same general laws, as previously shown in the experiments on frogs and fishes,[*] it might be expected that since chloroform and ether can be shown to pass off in the expired air, alcohol would also be exhaled in the same manner. Common experience, so far as the sense of smell is concerned, is in accordance with this view. Leibig, however, says,[†] "according to all the observations hitherto made, neither the expired air, nor the

---

[*] Med. Gaz., last vol., p. 622.
[†] Animal Chemistry, p. 239.

urine, contains any trace of alcohol, after indulgence in spirituous liquors." This, so far as I know, was true as regards the human subject, but Dr. Percy[*] had obtained alcohol by distilling the urine of a dog, to which he had given a fatal dose of it.

Feeling a strong conviction that alcohol must pass off in the breath, I have made many experiments during the last twelvemonths, with a view to detect it. At first, I caused the expired air, after spirit had been drunk, to pass, for an hour or longer, through a spiral tube, immersed in ice and salt, but did not succeed in detecting alcohol in the condensed water. A little reflection, however, made it evident that alcohol could only exist there in extremely minute quantities; for the spirit which had been taken, being equivalent only to two ounces of absolute alcohol, the inspired air would only be able to take up about a two-hundredth part as much vapour of alcohol as would saturate it, at the heat of the body; and it would be in vain to attempt to reduce the air to such a low temperature as would cause it to deposit any part of so relatively small an amount of vapour; in other words, the alcoholic dew-point of the air must be lower than the temperature of the ice and salt, and, consequently, all the spirit that could be arrested would be that which might be attracted by the small quantity of condensed water. By collecting together the water condensed from the breath in six different experiments, I succeeded, however, in obtaining spirit in a pure state, as will be detailed further on.

In the following experiments the same method was employed, as detailed above, for the detection of ether.

Exr. 62.—August 6th, 1850. Two ounces and a half of rectified spirit of wine, of 80 per cent., were diluted with rather less than a pint of water, and taken, with bread and butter, at supper-time. A slight feeling of inebriation was occasioned by it, but not sufficient to interfere, in the least, with the proper performance of the experiment. The air was afterwards taken in by the nostrils and breathed out by the mouth, through a wide tube communicating with a metal box containing a spiral arrangement, by which the air was

obliged to pass round several times. This box was surrounded with ice. The air was conducted next, by a glass tube half an inch wide, to the bottom of a bottle containing half a fluid ounce of sulphuric acid. The object of condensing the moisture of the breath, in the metal box, was to prevent its diluting the sulphuric acid beyond the point at which it ceases to decompose alcohol when heated. The expired air was, in this maner, passed through the sulphuric acid for thirty-five minutes. Care was taken that no air coming from the stomach by eructation should pass into the apparatus. Two and a half fluid drachms of clear water were condensed in the metal box. The following morning, the sulphuric acid was put into a small retort, communicating with a gas receiver over water, and heated with the flame of a spirit lamp. The acid was rendered quite black, and 5·1 cubic inches of gas were obtained, of which 2·6 cubic inches consisted of air from the retort. The receiver being transferred to the mercurial trough, and a little solution of potassa introduced, 1·65 cubic inches were absorbed. The jar being inverted, and a light applied to its mouth, the remaining contents took fire, the flame gradually descending in the jar to the surface of the mercury. The quantity of inflammable gas was 0·85 cubic inch.

Exr. 63.—Another night the same quantity of rectified spirit was taken, in the same manner, and the expired air passed through the spiral box and the sulphuric acid as before. Six fluid drachms of acid were employed this time, and the process of breathing through it was continued for an hour. Two and a half drachms of water were again condensed in the metal box, and the acid was increased in bulk by rather more than half a drachm. The sulphuric acid was next morning placed in a retort and heated. It was turned black, and six cubic inches of gas were obtained, two of which consisted of air from the retort. Solution of potassa absorbed 3·45 cubic inches of carbonic acid gas, and the remaining contents of the receiver burnt with a slight explosion, on a light being applied. The inflammable gas did not amount to more than 0·55 cubic inch.

Exr. 64.—The same quantity of rectified spirit was taken at night on another occasion, and the expired air passed for an hour through sulphuric acid in

[*] Prize Thesis "On the Presence of Alcohol in the Brain," &c.

the same way as before. The quantity of acid employed this time was a fluid ounce. On the following morning six drachms of the acid were heated in a small retort: they were rendered quite black, and somewhat viscid. 4·85 cubic inches of gas were obtained in the receiver, of which 1·8 cubic inch consisted of air from the retort; potash absorbed 0·6 cubic inch; 0·85 cubic inch of the remainder was transferred into a small jar, to the mouth of which a taper was applied, when the contents burnt for a little time with a bluish flame. To the residue in the receiver 3·8 cubic inches of oxygen were added, and a portion of the mixture was introduced into the eudiometer. As it did not explode with the electric spark, a small quantity of pure hydrogen gas was added, when an explosion was effected with the following result:—

Hydrogen	3·0
Oxygen, &c. . . .	32·0
Total	35·0
After explosion . .	27·0
Diminution	8·0

being a loss of 3·5 more than occasioned by the hydrogen.

Solution of potassa being agitated in the remaining 27 parts, they were diminished to 19; showing an absorption of 8 parts of carbonic acid. The loss of volume was consequently very nearly half as great as the quantity of carbonic acid gas produced by the explosion; and therefore the inflammable gas under examination was carbonic oxide, the amount of which was just one-fourth of the mixed gas introduced into the eudiometer. It is evident on calculation that nearly 1·8 cubic inch of carbonic oxide must have been expelled from the retort, and that this and the carbonic acid were the only gases evolved by the sulphuric acid.

The decomposition which the alcohol, absorbed from the expired air, undergoes in the sulphuric acid is the same as that undergone by the ether in the experiments previously detailed.

Exp. 65.—The water condensed in the metal box, surrounded with ice in the above three experiments, and in three others not related, amounted together to two ounces. It was placed in a retort, and about three drachms were distilled. This product was placed in a smaller retort, and about twenty minims were distilled into a small test tube. Dry carbonate of potassa was added to this till it would dissolve no more. In a little time, a layer of clear spirit, about the tenth of an inch in thickness, floated on the top of the solution of potash. A piece of asbestos being dipped in this, it burnt with a blue flame. A very little powdered camphor was dropped into a small tube, drawn at one end to a capillary point. This point being brought in contact with the liquid floating on the solution of potash, a little of it rose by capillary attraction, and was observed to dissolve the camphor within. On blowing at the other end of the tube, a minute drop of solution of camphor was forced out, and received on a piece of glass, when the spirit immediately evaporated, leaving a coating of camphor. These tests leave no doubt of the presence of alcohol. The process used in this experiment is similar to that employed by Dr. Percy for the detection of alcohol in the brain and other organs.

Exp. 66.—Two and a half fluid ounces of rectified spirit, of 80 per cent., were diluted with water, and taken at suppertime. The air was afterwards inspired for fifty minutes by the nostrils, and expired by the mouth, through a glass tube which dipped into three ounces of water contained in a bottle. Next morning the water was put into a retort, and about three drachms were distilled, which were put into a smaller retort, and about twenty minims were distilled into a small test tube. On carbonate of potassa being added in excess, a thin layer of clear liquid floated on the surface. This was proved to be alcohol; for a little bit of asbestos being moistened in it, burnt with a blue flame, and it dissolved camphor in the way described in the former experiment.

Whilst the above experiments show that alcohol is exhaled in the breath after it has been taken into the stomach, a little consideration will prove that only a small part of it can be excreted in this manner. When there are two ounces of alcohol in the blood, the air which reaches the lungs can only take up, as stated before, about a two-hundredth part as much as would saturate it at the temperature of the blood. At this rate, a person breathing the usual amount of air would only exhale about twelve minims of alcohol in an hour;

consequently, if it had to pass off entirely in the expired air, its effects would continue for a very much longer period than they do; and, since alcohol can hardly be detected in the other excretions, it must be decomposed in the system into fresh products.

I have assumed from the first that the speedy subsidence of the narcotism caused by chloroform and ether, in comparison with that from alcohol and other narcotics, depends on the volatility of the former substances, which allows of their ready exit by the expired air. Indeed, the effects of these medicines usually subside in the period which a calculation founded on this view would assign to them. It was previously estimated, for instance, that twenty-four minims of chloroform are contained in the blood of an adult of average size in a state of very complete insensibility; this being about one-twenty-eighth part as much as the blood would dissolve. The inhalation being now discontinued, the fresh air which reaches the air cells will abstract from the blood nearly one-twenty-eighth part as much as it can hold in suspension at the temperature of 100°; and as each hundred cubic inches of air, when saturated at 100°, contains 43·3 cubic inches of vapour of chloroform, 43 3÷28=1·54 cubic inches, or 1·48 minims, will be the quantity removed by the first hundred cubic inches of air which reaches the air-cells. It has been shown that about half the inspired air gets as far as the air-cells; and, supposing the patient to be breathing 400 cubic inches in the minute, 200 cubic inches would act in the removal of the vapour. In this manner it would take two minutes and a half to reduce the quantity of chloroform from 24 to 18 minims, and the narcotism from the fourth to the third degree; after which the effects would diminish more slowly, and in three and a half minutes longer the narcotism would have diminished to the second degree. Then, as the air would only take up about one-fifty-sixth part as much as it would hold, in about five minutes longer we might expect the return of consciousness; and the slight dizziness or confusion which might remain would subside still more gradually. The above statement expresses pretty well what usually occurs when the inhalation has been kept up for a little

time. Children recover from the effects of chloroform more rapidly, on account of their quicker circulation and respiration. Old people, on the other hand, more slowly, for the opposite reason. When insensibility is produced in the course of two minutes for a short operation, and the inhalation is not repeated, the effects of the vapour subside more quickly than stated above; because, at the same time that the chloroform is passing off by the lungs, it is also escaping from the main current of the circulation, by permeating the coats of the small vessels, and diffusing itself in the tissues, and thus allowing the brain to resume its functions.

Ether is more volatile than chloroform; but being also much more soluble, the relative quantity absorbed into the system is so much greater, as to more than compensate for the superior volatility; and consequently the effects of ether subside somewhat more slowly than those of chloroform, the ether taking rather longer to pass off in the expired air.

It follows as a necessary consequence of this mode of excretion of a vapour, that, if its exhalation by the breath could in any way be stopped, its narcotic effects ought to be much prolonged. The following experiments show that such is the case:—

EXP. 67.—About 750 cubic inches of oxygen gas were introduced into a balloon of thin membrane, varnished with solution of Indian rubber in turpentine. The balloon was attached to one of the apertures of the spiral box which forms part of the ether inhaler I employ, and which was used for condensing the moisture in the experiments on alcohol previously detailed. Four ounces of solution of potassa were put into the inhaler, and to its other opening was attached a tube, connected with a facepiece without valves.* After inhaling as much chloroform as I could without being rendered unconscious, I immediately began to breathe the oxygen from and to the balloon, and over the solution of potassa. In this way the vapour exhaled in the breath had, the greater part of it, to be re-inspired. This process was continued for ten

* I used the same arrangement in giving oxygen gas last year, at the request of Dr. Wilson, to a cholera patient in St. George's Hospital. The patient, who was in a state of collapse, was not saved or relieved by it.

minutes, during which time the feeling of narcotism subsided very little, and it passed off very slowly afterwards, about half an hour elapsing before it was quite gone.

The oxygen was used, in this and the following experiments, to allow of respiration being continued for some time from the balloon without employing such an amount of air as would take up a great deal of the vapour. As there was air both in the lungs and inhaler at the beginning of the experiment, the oxygen was not breathed unmixed with nitrogen. The solution of caustic potash was employed for the purpose of absorbing the carbonic acid gas generated by respiration as the air passed to and fro over a large extent of its surface.

Exp. 68.—On another day the same quantity of oxygen and solution of potassa were employed, and fifteen minims of chloroform were placed in the spiral inhaler, in a small glass vessel, which prevented its mixing with the solution of potassa. I then began to breathe as in the former experiment, and continued to do so for fifteen minutes. The effects of the chloroform were gradually induced during the first three minutes, causing a considerable feeling of narcotism, but not producing unconsciousness. After the end of three minutes, the feeling of narcotism remained stationary till twelve minutes had elapsed, and during the last three minutes it very slightly diminished. The experiment was discontinued on account of a feeling of want of breath. It was half an hour longer before the effects of the chloroform were altogether removed.

Exp. 69.—The oxygen and solution of potassa were employed as before, and two and a half fluid drachms of ether were put into the inhaler, with the potash. The oxygen was breathed to and fro over the potash for twenty minutes. The effects of the ether were rapidly developed during the first three minutes, but not amounting to loss of consciousness. From this time, the influence of the ether remained nearly the same to the end of the experiment, and afterwards subsided very gradually.

The effects of the small quantity of chloroform and ether inhaled in these experiments would have passed off in three or four minutes, if the exhaled vapour had been allowed to diffuse itself in the air in the usual way.

The amount of carbonic acid absorbed by the potassa was determined, and will be given in the next communication, as it forms a separate branch of the inquiry into the action of narcotic vapours.

———

PART XVI.

Experiments to determine the amount of Carbonic Acid Gas excreted under the influence of Chloroform—of Ether.— Diminution of Carbonic Acid caused by Alcohol.—Chloroform, Ether, &c., produce their effects by diminishing Oxidation in the system, without necessarily combining with oxygen themselves.—Proofs of this view.

In order to ascertain with accuracy the quantity of carbonic acid gas excreted by animals whilst under the influence of chloroform and ether, I employ some apparatus similar to part of that used by MM. V. Regnault and J. Reiset in their chemical researches on the respiration of animals.[*]

The accompanying engraving will assist to give a correct idea of the apparatus. The animal to be experimented on having been placed in a large glass jar, the latter is covered with a lid, padded on its under surface with an India rubber cushion, to make it fit accurately. In this lid there are three apertures. One of them serves for introducing the chloroform or ether, and can be closed by a brass mount; the others are connected, by means of tubes of vulcanized India rubber, to a potash apparatus, consisting of two glass vessels with an opening at each end, connected together at the lower part by means of another elastic tube. The solution of potash employed is diluted with sufficient pure water to make it fill one of the vessels; and as these vessels are made to move up and down during the experiment, by means of a cord passing over pullies, the solution of potassa is moved alternately from one vessel to the other, its place being occupied by air from the jar, which is returned back again as the vessel descends and becomes again filled with the liquid. As the tube from one of the potash vessels is continuous with

———

[*] Annales de Chimie et de Physique, 1849.

G

one which descends nearly to the bottom of the jar containing the animal subjected to experiment, air is alternately withdrawn and returned at its upper and lower part. A constant circulation of air thus takes place, and the carbonic acid gas becomes absorbed soon after it is given off from the lungs.

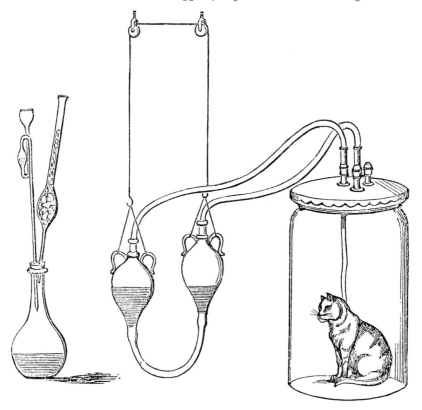

To determine the quantity of carbonic acid gas taken up by the solution of potassa, it is first put into a flask and boiled, to expel the chloroform or ether it may have absorbed. The flask is afterwards closed with a stopper, perforated for the admission of a safety tube, and a tube containing chloride of calcium.* The whole is then carefully weighed, together with a bottle containing rather more dilute sulphuric acid than is sufficient to saturate the solution of potassa. The acid is introduced gradually through the safety tube, and the contents of the flask heated to the boiling point, in order to expel the whole of the carbonic acid gas from the liquid. By making aspiration through the chloride of calcium tube, the whole of the carbonic acid is removed from the flask, its place becoming occupied by fresh atmospheric air, which enters through the other tube. When the contents of the flask

have cooled to the temperature at which the previous weighing took place, the apparatus is again carefully weighed, and the loss of weight shows the quantity of dry carbonic gas expelled. On deducting from this the small quantity of carbonic acid known to have been contained in the solution of potassa employed, the remainder shows the quantity which has been absorbed by it during the experiment.

Exp. 70.—On December 18th, 1850, a rabbit, weighing four pounds, was placed in a jar holding 1,600 cubic inches, and allowed to remain for half an hour, the potash apparatus above described being kept in motion during this time. The rabbit was very quiet during this part of the experiment.

The potash vessels having been emptied and replenished, and the rabbit having been removed for a few minutes for the ventilation of the jar, it was put in again, and twenty-five grains of chloroform were introduced through the

* See figure at the left side of the engraving.

aperture in the cover. The vessels containing the solution of potassa were kept moving up and down, as before. The rabbit moved about briskly on the introduction of the chloroform, and continued to do so for six minutes, after which it lay apparently asleep, but started spontaneously, now and then, as if in a disturbed dream. On its removal it showed signs of sensibility when touched, but appeared quite unconscious.

After being out of the jar for five minutes, and the jar having been well ventilated in the meantime, the rabbit was put in again, in much the same state as when removed. It remained for half an hour, sleeping the greater part of the time, but had almost recovered from the effects of the chloroform on its removal. The potash apparatus was in action as before.

The solution of potassa employed in the different parts of the experiment was analysed, with the precautions before described, and gave the following results:—

The quantity of carbonic acid gas absorbed in the first part of the experiment, before the exhibition of chloroform, was 6·80 grains. In the second part of the experiment, during the inhalation of chloroform, 2·78 grains were absorbed; and 2·85 grains after the inhalation, whilst the rabbit was gradually recovering.

EXP. 71.—On December 21st, 1850, a young dog, weighing eight pounds, was placed in the jar holding 1,600 cubic inches, and allowed to remain half an hour, the potash apparatus being kept moving, as in the previous experiment. The dog whined and turned round occasionally, but did not make much muscular effort.

The dog having been removed for a few minutes in order to ventilate the jar, was put in again, and twenty-five minims (thirty-six grains) of chloroform were introduced. The potash apparatus, which had been replenished, was moved up and down as before. On the introduction of the chloroform the dog made violent efforts to escape, and his muscular exertions continued, when they were no longer directed by consciousness, till he sank down apparently insensible at the end of about eight minutes. The head and limbs, however, continued to be moved occasionally during the remainder of the half hour. On his re-

moval from the jar the dog yelped, but his muscles were quite flaccid, and he lay for a time where he was placed, and afterwards recovered gradually.

The solution of potassa employed in the half hour just before the chloroform, was found to have absorbed 10·1 grains of carbonic acid gas, whilst that employed for the same period with the chloroform had absorbed only 4·8 grains.

EXP. 72.—On January 19, 1851, a cat about half-grown was placed in a jar holding 920 cubic inches, and allowed to remain for half an hour whilst the potash apparatus was in operation, as in the other experiments. The cat made occasional efforts to get out of the jar.

A few minutes after its removal from the jar, the cat was put in again, and twenty grains of chloroform were introduced through the aperture in the cover. The potash apparatus, having been replenished, was kept in motion, as before. On the introduction of the chloroform the cat made violent efforts to get out. In two or three minutes it became unconscious; but it continued to move involuntarily until five minutes had elapsed, when it sank down in a state of insensibility. During the remaining twenty-five minutes of the experiment the breathing was quick, and much deeper than natural. The cat was quite insensible to pricking and pinching on its removal.

The solution of potassa employed just before the chloroform was given absorbed 5·7 grains of carbonic acid gas; whilst that used during the time that the chloroform was exhibited, absorbed but 2·0 grains.

EXP. 73.—On Feb. 17, 1851, a cat weighing four pounds and a half was placed in the jar holding 1600 cubic inches, and kept there for half an hour. It sat very quietly the whole time. A few minutes afterwards it was put into the same jar again, and eighteen grains of chloroform were introduced by the aperture in the lid. The cat moved about somewhat during the first seven or eight minutes, but it lay sleeping the remainder of the half-hour: it was not insensible on its removal, but inclined to sleep when not disturbed. The cat, having been removed for a few minutes to ventilate the jar, was put in again, and twenty-seven grains of chloroform were introduced. The cat had in a great measure recovered from the effects of the former dose of chloroform during its removal: it attempted to escape on the fresh chloroform being introduced, but soon became quiet and apparently insensible. At the end of half an hour the solution of potassa was changed, without removing the animal from the jar. Chloroform was now added by ten minims at a time, about every ten minutes, till the cat was killed. It died very gradually at the end of three-quarters of an hour. The breathing became very feeble, and intermitted, for long intervals before death took place, and there were no gaspings.

The potash apparatus was in operation during the experiment, and the analysis of the solution of potass gave the following results:—

Carbonic acid gas excreted in half an hour, just before the chloroform, 7·7 grains.

In half an hour, with eighteen grains of chloroform in the jar, 5·7 grains.

In the same time, with twenty-seven grains of chloroform, 4·9 grains.

During the last three-quarters of an hour, 7·1 grains, which is at the rate of 4·7 grains for half an hour.

It will be observed that the quantity of carbonic acid gas excreted under the influence of chloroform was considerably less in all the above experiments than it had been just before; and, in the last experiment, it will be remarked that the excretion of carbonic acid kept diminishing as the narcotism increased; whilst in Exp. 70 it increased somewhat during the last stage of the experiment, whilst the effects of the chloroform were subsiding.

It would not be easy to make correct experiments for ascertaining the amount of carbonic acid gas excreted by patients whilst under the influence of chloroform; and my inquiries on this point in the human subject have been confined to such experiments as I could conduct on myself whilst slightly affected by the vapour.

In two experiments related in the last part of this series of papers,* in which oxygen gas was breathed to and fro over solution of potassa, whilst under the partial influence of chloroform, the amount of carbonic acid absorbed by the potash was determined in the manner described above, for comparison with that absorbed in experiments conducted in a similar manner a little time before the chloroform was inhaled. The quantity of carbonic acid was diminished by the chloroform, as is shown in the following table:—In Exp. 67, for instance, 42 grains of carbonic acid gas were absorbed by the potash whilst breathing oxygen for ten minutes, before the chloroform had been inhaled, and only 33 grains during the same period, just after the inhalation of chloroform. A similar diminution of the amount of carbonic acid took place in Exp. 68.

In the subsequent experiments enumerated in the table, the air was inspired by the nostrils and expired by the mouth, through a glass tube which conveyed it through a solution of potassa placed in two Woulfe's bottles. The ex-

No. of Exp.	Date of Exp.	Duration of Exp.		Carbonic Acid.		Carb. Acid per min.	
		Before Chlorm.	With Chlorm.	Before Chlorm.	With Chlorm.	Before Chlorm.	With Chlorm.
67	Sep. 3, 1850.	10 min.	10 min.	42·0 grs.	33·0 grs.	4·20 grs.	3·30 grs.
68	Sep. 19, „	15 „	15 „	73·0 „	46·0 „	4·86 „	3·06 „
74	Oct. 28, „	10 „	10 „	23·0 „	20·5 „	23.0 „	2·05 „
75	Oct. 30, „	20 „	20 „	57·0 „	53·0 „	2·85 „	2·65 „
76	Oct. 31, „	15 „	15 „	42·0 „	36·5 „	2·80 „	2·43 „
77	Mar. 18, 1851.	20 „	20 „	43·0 „	37·5 „	2·17 „	1·87 „
Mean quantity of carbonic acid per minute.						3·19 grs.	2·56 grs.

* MEDICAL GAZETTE, last vol. p. 753.

periments were made at ten or eleven o'clock in the evening, after sitting quietly for two or three hours. The breath was passed through the solution of potassa before inhaling, and then through a similar solution, after inhaling as much chloroform, for three or four minutes, as could be taken without causing unconsciousness. An inspiration of chloroform was also taken, now and then, during the remainder of the experiment, to prevent the effects of the vapour from altogether subsiding.

Soon after the introduction of the inhalation of ether, I made some observations on the amount of carbonic acid gas exhaled from the lungs under its influence, by passing the expired air through lime water, when I found the quantity to be diminished.* The following more recent experiments on animals have been attended with a similar result.

Exp. 78.—On Dec. 15, 1850, a rabbit, weighing four pounds, was kept in a jar, of the capacity of 1600 cubic inches, for forty minutes, the potash apparatus, before described, being in motion all the time. The rabbit was perfectly quiet. Soon afterwards, the rabbit was put into the jar again, and forty grains of ether were introduced, which did not cause insensibility, but only inebriation. The rabbit remained in a position between sitting and lying, being able to hold its head up. It was removed at the end of forty minutes.

Twenty minutes after its removal, when the effects of the ether had almost altogether gone off, the rabbit was a third time placed in the jar, for the space of forty minutes.

The analysis of the potash employed in the first part of the experiment, before the ether, yielded 12·6 grains of carbonic acid The carbonic acid given off during the inhalation of ether was not correctly determined, owing to an accident ; but that employed in the third part of the experiments yielded 10·8 grains, showing a notable diminution, although the effects of the ether on the animal had almost ceased to be perceptible

Exp. 79.—In March, 1851, two pigeons were placed for twenty minutes in a jar holding 670 cubic inches.

They stood still the whole time. A few minutes after their removal they were put into the jar again, and sixty grains of ether were introduced, at short intervals, by a few grains at a time. The pigeons became gradually insensible, and at the end of eight minutes were lying on the side. They showed no signs of sensibility when removed at the end of twenty minutes, but lay where they were placed. After being out for three minutes, they were put into the jar again, as they were beginning to evince signs of returning sensibility. In ten minutes more they were able to stand, but they were not fully recovered, when they were removed, at the end of twenty minutes.

The potash apparatus was in action, as in the previous experiments. The solution of potassa employed in the first part of the experiment absorbed 6·1 grains of carbonic acid; that employed in the second part absorbed 3·6 grains ; and that employed in the last part of the experiment, whilst the effects of the ether were subsiding, absorbed 4·4 grains.

The late Dr. Prout discovered, nearly forty years ago, that fermented and spirituous liquors diminish the amount of carbonic acid given off from the lungs. He summed up the result of his experiments on this point in the following words :—"Alcohol, in every state, and in every quantity, uniformly lessens, in a greater or less degree, the quantity of carbonic acid gas elicited, according to the quantity and circumstances under which it is taken."* Dr. Prout's experiments were confined to the proportion of carbonic acid gas in the expired air. A recent German author has extended his inquiries to the quantity exhaled in a given time, and he finds that both the proportions in the expired air and the quantity excreted per minute are diminished during the action of alcohol. He also finds that the total amount of every one of the constituents of the urine is lessened, under the same circumstances.†

The diminution of the amount of carbonic acid formed in the system

---

* See Report of Westminster Med. Soc. in Med. Gaz., Feb. 26, 1847.

* Ann. Phil. vol. ii. p. 336.
† Beiträge zur Heilkunde nach eigenen Untersuchungen von Friedr. Wilh. Böcker. Crefeld, 1849. I am indebted to the kindness of Dr. Bence Jones for the knowledge of this work.

under the influence of chloroform, ether, and alcohol, taken in conjunction with a circumstance shown in a former paper, that the chloroform and ether are exhaled unchanged from the blood, assist to prove a view of their modus operandi which I suggested with respect to ether, early in 1847.* That view may be stated as follows.

Chloroform, ether, and similar substances, when present in the blood in certain quantities, have the effect of limiting those combinations between the oxygen of the arterial blood and the tissues of the body which are essential to sensation, volition, and, in short, all the animal functions. The substances modify, and in larger quantities arrest, the animal functions, in the same way, and by the same power, that they modify and arrest combustion, the slow oxidation of phosphorus, and other kinds of oxidation unconnected with the living body, when they are mixed in certain quantities with the atmospheric air.

This explanation is probably applicable to the action of all narcotics whatever, but is here applied only to the class considered in these papers, namely, the volatile narcotic substances not containing nitrogen, or those substances whose power was found to be in the inverse ratio of their solubility in water and the serum of the blood.

The circumstances which appear to my mind fully to establish the above stated theory of the operation of chloroform and similar bodies, are enumerated in the following propositions :—

1. Sensation, motion, thought, and indeed all the strictly animal functions, are as closely connected with certain processes of oxidation going on in the body, as the light and heat of flame are connected with the oxidation of the burning materials.

2. The diminution of the amount of carbonic acid gas excreted by the lungs under the influence of chloroform, ether, and alcohol, shows that the processes of oxidation going on in the body are lessened, for the amount of carbonic acid given off has a pretty close relation to the quantity of oyxgen consumed.

3. The diminution of temperature in animals under the influence of chloroform and ether, alluded to in an early part of these papers, also shows that the proceesses of oxidation which take place in the body are diminished, since the development of animal heat has been shown, by Edwards and others, to have a constant relation to the quantity of oxygen which is consumed in respiration.

4. The venous blood in patients under the influence of chloroform or ether is less dark in colour than in the normal state; indicating that those changes in the blood which take place in the systemic capillary circulation are diminished.

5. The lessened quantity of all the constituents of the urine, observed by Böcker, from the effects of alcohol, also shows that oxidation is diminished.

6. The diminished oxidation is not owing to the combination of the narcotic substance with the oxygen of the arterial blood; for in the first place, the chloroform and ether, as well as part of the alcohol, have been shown to escape unaltered in the breath; in the second place, the quantity of material, in the case of chloroform, capable of combining with oxygen, is altogether insufficient so to appropriate the oxygen; and in the third place, to increase the amount of oxygen in the respired air does not prevent the action of the narcotics.

7. The different parts of the nervous system lose their power under the influence of the narcotics we are considering, in the same order as in asphyxia— the privation of oxygen, as was observed by M. Flourens with respect to ether, in 1847.*

8. The muscular irritability, which continues for a short time after death, depends on the action of a little oxygen still remaining in the system; and this irritability can be at once extinguished by chloroform, ether, or alcohol, in proportion rather larger than is necessary to cause death. When the muscular irritability is thus extinguished, postmortem rigidity comes on almost immediately, and lasts for an unusually long time, if the narcotic employed is prevented from evaporating.

9. The vapours of volatile narcotic substances have the property, when mixed with the air, of retarding, and, in larger quantity, of arresting, that form of oxidation which constitutes ordinary

---

* See MED. GAZ. vol. xxxix. p. 383.

* Gazette des Hôpitaux, 20 Mars, 1847.

combustion; and their power in preventing combustion generally bears a direct relation to their narcotic strength.

10. Many of these same vapours have the property of preventing the slow oxidation of phosphorus, which renders it luminous in the dark, as was discovered by Prof. Graham; and their effects, in this respect, have a general relation to their narcotic power.

11. The putrefaction of animal substances consists, on its commencement at least, of a process of oxidation; and the numerous class of substances we are considering all have the property of preventing putrefaction, their antiseptic power having generally a direct relation to their narcotic properties.

12. The reduction of the temperature of the body, by exposure to cold, diminishes the consumption of oxygen, and causes symptoms very nearly resembling the effects of a narcotic.

The second and sixth of the above propositions have already been fully considered, and the remainder will receive further consideration in my next paper.

ON

NARCOTISM

BY THE

INHALATION OF VAPOURS.

BY

JOHN SNOW, M.D.

LICENTIATE OF THE ROYAL COLLEGE OF PHYSICIANS.

PARTS XVII. AND XVIII.

From the London Medical Gazette for December 1851.

LONDON:

PRINTED BY WILSON AND OGILVY,

57, SKINNER STREET, SNOWHILL.

1852.

PART XVII.

FOR a length of time after the changes which are effected in the air by respiration were discovered, it was generally believed that the carbonic acid was formed in the lungs, by the union of the oxygen of the air with carbon contained in the blood; and the phenomena of asphyxia were thought to be occasioned by the direct action of some form or combination of carbon which ought to have been excreted. Experiments by Edwards, and others, on the respiration of animals in hydrogen gas, and especially the beautiful experiments of Professor Magnus on the blood, clearly proved, however, what many physiologists had believed from the first, — that the oxygen of the air is absorbed (along with some nitrogen) and circulates with the arterial blood, combining with carbon in the systemic capillary circulation, and thus forming the carbonic acid which is exhaled from the blood in its passage through the lungs. Asphyxia is simply due to the want of oxygen in the arterial blood; for, although there is a little carbonic acid gas present in this blood during the more ordinary forms of asphyxia, yet the same symptoms occur to animals placed in hydrogen or nitrogen gas, although the carbonic acid gas in the blood is then exhaled. The presence of oxygen in the blood seems absolutely necessary to the performance of the animal functions — so necessary that none of them can continue an instant without it. Animals live, it is true, for a short time after they are deprived of air, but a little consideration shows that they live only by virtue of the oxygen which is contained in their bodies, and that when this is consumed life no longer continues. The length of time which animals live after they are deprived of air is in the inverse ratio of the activity of their functions, and Dr. W. F. Edwards has shown[*] that animals of cold blood, as reptiles and fishes, die of asphyxia, nearly as quickly as animals of warm blood, when they are placed in water deprived of air, and of a temperature of about 100° Fah. The increase of heat quickens the changes taking place in the body, as the same author has proved by distinct experiments: the oxygen dissolved in the fluids of the animal is soon appropriated, and life is then extinct. Animals of cold blood can also be quickly killed at the ordinary temperature by the rapid absorption of agents, such as the vapour of ether, which have the undoubted power of arresting oxidation out of the body, and when present in the blood in sufficient quantity, have the effect of preventing the oxygen it contains from any longer entering into combination. The experiments of Dr. Kay[†] show that venous blood has some power of supporting the functions of the brain, and the irritability of the muscles when injected into the arteries, but this depends on some free oxygen it contains; for the analyses of Magnus have proved that arterial blood is only deprived of part of its oxygen by passing once through the systemic capillaries.

The relation between asphyxia and narcotism is this — that in asphyxia there is an absence of oxygen, whilst in narcotism the oxygen is present, but is prevented from acting by the influence of the narcotic. With this close affinity between asphyxia and narcotism, as regards their intimate nature, there is, as might be expected, a great similarity in the phenomena of the two conditions. The different parts of the nervous centres lose their power, under the influence of ether and chloroform, in the

---

[*] De l'Influence des Agens Physiques sur la Vie.

[†] The Physiology, Pathology, and Treatment of Asphyxia, p. 193.

same order as in asphyxia. The action of the heart continues in asphyxia after the muscles of respiration have ceased to contract, and this is the case under the effects of chloroform, alcohol, ether, and probably all narcotics, when they are absorbed in a gradual and uniform manner. For, as the muscular contractions of a peristaltic character, which are under the influence of the ganglionic system of nerves, can go on with a smaller amount of oxygen than those which are dependent on the cerebro-spinal system, so it requires a larger quantity of the narcotic to arrest them. During sudden asphyxia of robust subjects by privation of air, there are generally convulsions after the loss of consciousness, and there is likewise usually an amount of muscular rigidity and contraction approaching to convulsions when insensibility is quickly induced by chloroform or ether, in muscular persons or robust animals. By gradually inducing narcotism these contractions can be avoided, and in like manner, when asphyxia is slowly induced by vitiation of a limited supply of air, convulsions are not induced. The impediment offered to the absorption of oxygen in the lungs during bronchitis is sometimes accompanied by delirium not unlike that caused by a narcotic, and occasionally coma is met with. The state of the fœtus in utero—just able to perform a few languid movements of its limbs—resembles very much the sleep caused by a narcotic. At this time it receives only a limited supply of oxygen at second hand through the placenta; but on being born, no sooner has it taken one or two free inspirations, than it exhibits an amount of activity and strength which would be fatal to the mother did it possess it whilst in the womb.

With all these points of resemblance between narcotism and asphyxia, it might perhaps be asked why a limitation of the supply of air, or in other words a partial asphyxia, might not be resorted to instead of a narcotic to prevent the pain of operations. The answer must probably be sought in the circumstance remarked by all the observers of the phenomena of asphyxia, that the blood becomes arrested at the pulmonary capiliaries, when oxygen is no longer admitted into the air-cells of the lungs. On this account insensibility cannot be induced by means of asphyxia, without causing congestion of the lungs, and great distress of the respiration.

In a profound state of narcotism the symptoms often exactly resemble those of apoplexy. In both conditions there is a partial suspension of the process of oxidation on which the functions of the brain depend; but this impediment to the natural process of oxidation arises from a different cause in the two cases. In narcotism it is due to the presence of the narcotic substance in the blood, which retards oxidation, as we shall presently see, by a kind of counter affinity for the oxygen: in apoplexy it depends on more or less complete interruption to the circulation of the blood. For the constant action between the oxygen of the arterial blood and the brain, there is obviously required a never-ceasing current of blood; and when this is interrupted in any part of the brain, it is clear that there must be an interference with the process of oxidation; and it matters not whether the circulation be interfered with by pressure arising from effusion, by the occlusion of one or more of the arteries which cuts off part of the supply, or by such an amount of congestion from any cause that the current of the circulation is interrupted. According to these views it ought not to signify whether there is increased or diminished pressure in the cranium, or whether the quantity of blood in the brain is more or less than natural; but if the circulation is interrupted or greatly impeded, there ought to be the symptoms which arise from impeded oxidation. Such indeed is the fact; we meet with the same symptoms in very different physical conditions of the contents of the cranium, and the question of bleeding and the application of other remedies cannot be decided by the cerebral symptoms alone, without the consideration of other particulars.

The circulation through the capillaries of the brain is undoubtedly sometimes retarded under the influence of narcotics; but this is the consequence and not the cause of the impeded functions of the brain. For, as was first pointed out by Professor Alison, the functions of the various organs of the body are accompanied by a force which aids the capillary circulation; and on the function of any organ being interrupted, the circulation through it is retarded, as s seen in the most striking manner in the lungs during asphyxia. There is this further difference also between narcotism and apoplexy, that the narcotic acts directly on all parts of the body as well as on the brain, whilst in apoplexy the remainder of the nervous system and the other organs of the body are only effected in a secondary manner.

In my last communication,* several experiments were detailed which shew that the quantity of carbonic acid evolved from the lungs is considerably diminished under the influence of ether and chloroform. This circumstance indicates diminished oxidation, for carbonic acid is the chief product of that process in the animal frame, and it bears a pretty close relation to the amount of oxygen consumed. Dr. Prout formerly showed that the quantity of carbonic acid produced in respiration was diminished after drinking alcoholic liquors, and alcohol very much resembles ether and chloroform in chemical constitution and physiological effects. Under the influence of this agent, alcohol, Böcker ascertained, as was noticed before, that the amount of every one of the constituents of the urine is diminished, and phosphoric acid and urea are important products of oxidation.

In some experiments detailed in the first part of these papers,† the temperature of animals was seen to diminish under the continued influence of ether and chloroform. This circumstance is also illustrative of the diminished oxidation that is taking place, for the experiments of Dr. W. F. Edwards‡ on animals of various species, at different periods in their life, and in different seasons of the year, show that the consumption of oxygen in respiration always bears a direct proportion to the evolution of animal heat.§

* See last vol. p. 622.
† MEDICAL GAZETTE, vol. xli. p. 850.
‡ Op. cit.
§ The cooling of animals, in Sir B. Brodie's experiments, when the circulation was kept up by artificial respiration, after they were reduced to a state of suspended animation by narcotics, gives support to the above views, allowance being made for the artificial condition of the animals. The other experiments of this eminent physiologist, in which animals were found to cool rapidly under similar circumstances, after removal of the brain, are not at all opposed to the view that animal heat results from the process of respiration, if we reflect that respiration, or oxidation, is essential to all the animal functions, and that the formation of phosphoric acid and urea are probably as much accompanied by the evolution of caloric, as is the formation of carbonic acid.

Gradual exposure to a lower temperature, as happens in the change of season from summer to winter, alters the constitution of many animals, causing them to consume more oxygen, and thus to develope more heat, and bear up against a colder season ; but other species, including some mammalia, as well as nearly all reptiles, are narcotised by the cold, and fall into a state of torpor in the winter, when the consumption of oxygen is reduced to a minimum. Cold air, or whatever abstracts the heat of the body, so as to make a considerable reduction in its temperature, is a true narcotic, and acts like other narcotics, by diminishing oxidation. Travellers in the arctic regions inform us that the symptoms produced by intense cold are sometimes not to be distinguished from intoxication by alcohol, except by the circumstance that no spirituous liquors can have been obtained. As regards its local effects, cold is probably the narcotic which has been longest known to the human species ; for its benumbing effects (ναρκόω, I benumb) make themselves felt, in the fingers at least, in most parts of the earth, at some season of the year. The local application of cold closely resembles that of chloroform and many other narcotics, in causing a slight amount of pain before sensibility is altogether abolished. Dr. James Arnott, who has given great attention to the local effects of graduated temperature in the treatment of various affections, has relieved neuralgic pains by the application of a mixture of salt and pounded ice, and has also rendered the surface of the body so insensible, that the introduction of setons, and other operations of a superficial nature, have been performed without pain. Dr. Arnott calls the process congelation; but the hardness which is produced in the part must depend on the solidification of the adipose substance ; for if the water which enters into the composition of the tissues were frozen, their intimate structure would be destroyed, and a slough would be the result.

The effects of ether and chloroform on the appearance of the blood agree perfectly with the view above given of their modus operandi. There is generally no alteration in the complexion of the patient, or in the colour of the mixed venous and arterial blood as it flows from a wound, so long as the inhalation is not pushed to the extent of embarrassing the respiration, and provided the patient is not holding his breath, on account of the pungency of the vapour, or a general state of rigidity which sometimes occurs for a minute or two; but when the blood which flows from the arteries and veins can be separately observed, whilst the patient is well under the influence of the narcotic, it is seen that the arterial blood is somewhat less florid, and the venous blood less dark than under ordinary circumstances. The lighter colour of the venous blood, which has been spoken of by Dr Gull, as well as by myself, points particularly to a diminution of oxidation in the systemic capillaries.

The phenomena attending the irritability which remains in the muscles for a longer or shorter time after death, and particularly the effect of narcotics on this irritability, accord exactly with the views above expressed. It can be shown, by the following amongst other reasons, that the muscular irritability depends on a little oxygen still remaining in the blood contained in the muscular tissue. Nysten* found that the injection of oxygen gas into the cavities of the heart increased the vigour and duration of the contractions. Sir B. Brodie states that, in dogs in which the circulation was kept up after death by artificial respiration, " there seemed to be actually an increased irritability of the voluntary muscles, continued not for a short time, but even for an hour and a half."† Nysten informs us‡ that the general result of his observations on the duration of the muscular irritability in animals of different classes, and of different orders of the same class, was in the inverse ratio of the muscular energy developed during life; and we previously saw, on the authority of Edwards, that this was just the ratio of duration of life under privation of air or asphyxia.

Chloroform, ether, alcohol, and probably all narcotics, have the power of suspending the muscular irritability. In a former paper of this series§ some experiments were related in which the irritability of the heart in frogs and rabbits was removed by the vapour of chloroform; and in two of the experiments the irritability was alternately allowed to recover by letting the chloroform evaporate, and then suspended again by a fresh exposure to the vapour. In one of these experiments the peristaltic action of the small intestine of a rabbit was arrested by the local action of chloroform. I have frequently stopped the quivering motion of the intercostal muscles, which is seen on opening the chest of an animal immediately after death, by blowing a little vapour of chloroform on them through a tube. On one of these occasions Dr. Sibson was present.

The following experiments show the action of chloroform, &c., on all the muscles of the body :—

Exp. 80.—A half-grown guinea-pig was made to inhale chloroform in a glass jar till it ceased to breathe. The chest was then opened, and a tube armed with a stop-cock was introduced into the aorta and tied. The heart was still contracting, and the muscles were very sensible to the shocks of an electro-magnetic apparatus. Fifteen minims of chloroform, and two drachms of tepid water, which had been agitated together till the chloroform was suspenced in minutes globules, were now injected. At the moment of injection the right anterior extremity and the two posterior extremities were stretched out, and the toes quivered. These limbs became quite rigid at the moment of the injection, as did also the neck and trunk of the animal. The left anterior extremity remained flexible. The wires of the battery were applied to the muscles of various parts of the body immediately after the injection, but no contractions could be excited, except in the left anterior extremity, and the muscles of the chest on the same side, which remained as irritable as before; the reason of this being that the injection had not entered the left subclavian artery. The heart ceased to act at the moment of the injection, and was afterwards quite insensible to the shocks of the battery.

Exp. 81.—A similar guinea-pig to the last was killed by the inhalation of ether, and was opened immediately after it ceased to breathe, whilst the heart was still acting. The tube was secured in the descending aorta, and two fluid drachms of sulphuric ether were injected. The posterior extremities were stretched

* Recherches Physiologiques, p. 335.
† Physiological Researches, 1851, p. 108.
‡ Opus cit. p. 355.
§ Vol. xlii. p. 415, 614.

out at the time of the injection, and there was a quivering motion of the toes. These extremities, together with the posterior half of the trunk, became instantly affected with post-mortem rigidity, and were totally insensible to the shocks of the electro-magnetic battery. The anterior extremities, and, indeed, all the anterior part of the body which had not been injected with ether, remained sensible to the shocks of the battery, and only became rigid between two and three hours after death. The heart ceased to act at the moment of the injection, some ether having been dropped on it from the syringe.

Exp. 82.—An ounce of rectified spirit of wine was injected into the aorta of a cat immediately after death from chloroform. There were muscular contractions at the moment of injection, but no contractions could be excited afterwards by mechanical irritation, although the muscles were very irritable just before, and were quivering when not touched. The heart, which was previously beating, also ceased to act. Post-mortem rigidity began to take place five minutes after the injection, and it still existed eight days afterwards.

Exp. 83.—A cat was killed by inhalation of chloroform, and three minutes after death three drachms of rectified spirit of wine, of 80 per cent., were mixed with three drachms of water, and injected into the descending aorta. The posterior extremities were stretched out at the moment of the injection, and almost immediately began to be rigid; and in less than ten minutes after the injection, the whole of the posterior half of the body was very rigid, whilst the anterior parts were quite flexible. An hour after death rigidity was commencing in the anterior extremities, and in half an hour more they and the neck were quite rigid. This cat was killed on Dec. 1st, 1850, and was kept in a room with a fire. The rigidity of the anterior half of the body began to subside at the end of a week, but that of the posterior extremities not till a fortnight had elapsed; and they were still quite fresh, although putrefaction was commencing in the chest and neck.

As absorption of vapour continues in the frog by its skin after the respiratory movements have ceased, it is not necessary to resort either to dissection or injection in them, as in mammalia, in order to cause the extinction of irri-

tability, and bring on the post-mortem rigidity. It can be induced in a very few minutes by exposure to the vapour of ether or chloroform, although, under ordinary circumstances, the muscles remain long irritable and flexible in these animals. In some interesting experiments lately detailed in the MEDICAL GAZETTE by Mr. W. F. Barlow,[*] that gentleman produced rigidity in a single limb of living frogs without much affecting the rest of the animal; he also observed what I had previously remarked,[†] that the setting in of rigidity in these animals is sometimes accompanied by a movement of the body.

The state which is called post-mortem rigidity appears to be the natural condition of muscle when no kind of change in its composition is taking place. As long as the feeble oxidation continues, which enables it to be irritable after death, it remains flaccid; but when this ceases, from want of oxygen, from reduction of temperature, from the counter affinity of a narcotic, or from exhaustion of the nutrient materials, the muscle becomes rigid, and remains so till a new kind of oxidation—that of putrefaction—commences, when it again becomes flaccid. Although the muscles, when affected with this kind of rigidity, are in a state of completely suspended animation, they are not always incapable of again living; for M. Brown Sequard has restored the irritability of the muscles of a dead guinea pig after they had been rigid from ten to twenty minutes, by making the blood of a living animal of the same species circulate in its vessels. Although reducing the temperature hastens rigidity, it is not essential to it; for I have seen a fœtus at the full term born in a state of complete rigor mortis.

In a former paper[‡] several proofs were given that chloroform and ether do not prevent oxidation in the system by themselves combining with the oxygen of the blood. Among these proofs were some experiments showing that the chloroform and ether are exhaled again unchanged from the blood as it circulates through the lungs. The paper of next week will contain an inquiry into the manner in which these narcotics act in limiting and preventing oxidation in the living frame.

---

* Page 713.
† MED. GAZ., vol. xlii. p. 415.

PART XVIII.

Antiseptic power of narcotics—Narcotic vapours and gases prevent ordinary combustion—They prevent the slow combustion of hydrogen by means of spongy platinum—They prevent the oxidation of phosphorus—Nature of the power by which narcotics prevent oxidation in the living body and out of it—Recapitulation.

DURING the last two years, whilst the investigations which I have been making respecting chloroform and ether, and publishing from time to time in the MEDICAL GAZETTE, have been directed more particularly to showing the *modus operandi* of these agents, M. Robin, of Paris, has been engaged in a like inquiry, and has arrived at similar conclusions, although his researches have been made in a different manner. His opinion was given at the Academy of Sciences to the following effect:—That the anæsthetic action of the vapour of ether or chloroform is the result of a state of asphyxia more or less complete; but that this kind of asphyxia is produced by these agents, when absorbed, protecting the blood in the capillary vessels against the action of the oxygen, in the same way that they protect a piece of flesh, or any other animal substance that is plunged into them, against the action of the same agent, oxygen, and thus prevent putrefaction.* M. Robin subsequently gave his views to the Academy in a more extended form. He stated that all substances which will preserve dead animal and vegetable matters against putrefaction are capable of acting as poisons to all organised beings, whether possessed of a nervous system or not; that the action is independent of their coagulating or not coagulating albumen; and that it consists in the power they have of protecting organised matters from slow combustion by moist oxygen. He stated that they diminish or completely interrupt the combustion according to the quantity; and that, in proportion to the dose, they are sedative medicines to animals, and asphyxiating poisons to all organised beings.*

The following are amongst the substances enumerated by M. Robin as having the properties in question:—Sulphuric ether, chloroform, benzin, Dutch liquid, hydriodic ether, acetic ether, naphtha, sulphuret of carbon, camphor, protochloride of carbon, carburet of nitrogen, hydrocyanic acid, and arsenic. The first seven of the above agents are amongst those whose narcotic effects I have described in the MEDICAL GAZETTE.

The antiseptic power of these and other substances is probably in direct proportion to their narcotic strength; at all events, I have ascertained that such is the case as regards chloroform, ether, and alcohol. A few drops of chloroform, when put into a bottle, form enough vapour to prevent putrefaction in a piece of flesh suspended in it; but it requires a larger quantity of ether, which is a less powerful narcotic, to produce a like effect. One part of ether, when mixed with nine or ten parts of water, preserves animal matters; but a larger proportion of alcohol is required for a like effect; and alcohol, as is well known, requires to be taken in much larger quantity than ether to cause insensibility. I have often observed the antiseptic powers of chloroform, even in the small quantity which suffices to cause the death of an animal, especially when it has been inhaled slowly, so that the tissues were intimately impregnated with it. For instance, the cat which formed the subject of Experiment 73 in a former paper,

---

* See Comptes Rendus, t. xxx. p. 52.

* Comptes Rendus, t. xxxi p. 383 ; and MED. GAZ. vol. xlvi. p. 590.

and which was killed with chloroform, was kept for sixteen days in a temperature between 50° and 60° Fahr., and, at the end of that time, the rigor mortis was only beginning to subside, and putrefaction had scarcely commenced.*

The substances which have the property of limiting and preventing oxidation in the living body, have also the property of limiting and preventing that kind of oxidation which constitutes ordinary combustion. If, for instance, as much ether as will make not less than about eight cubic inches of vapour be diffused through the air of a bottle or jar holding one hundred cubic inches, and a lighted taper be lowered into the vessel, it will be extinguished. The vapour of ether will take fire at the mouth of the bottle; but the taper will go out as it descends into the air mixed with vapour not in a state of combustion. Flame is extinguished also by the vapour of chloroform when in sufficient quantity, and by many other vapours and gases. Sir Humphry Davy, whose investigations on flame resulted in the discovery of the safety-lamp, thought at first that the power of preventing combustion in these instances depended on the cooling power of the gas employed as a diluent; but, on making experiments with various gases, he found that some other cause or causes existed. Olefiant gas had a much greater effect in preventing the

explosion of oxygen and hydrogen by the electric spark than any of the other gases employed by Sir H. Davy, and this gas is a more powerful narcotic than carbonic acid, or any of the others he used, except sulphuretted hydrogen (which probably acts in a different manner from ordinary narcotics), for I have found that olefiant gas causes immediate insensibility in birds, when mixed with the air in the proportion of one part to ten.

Dr. Henry, and Professor Graham,* have ascertained that a number of gases have the effect of preventing the slow combination which takes place between oxygen and hydrogen with the aid of spongy platinum, and that the relative power of the various gases is nearly the same in this instance as when the electric spark is employed, olefiant gas being the most powerful.

Professor Graham discovered† that a number of vapours, as well as gases, have the property, when mixed with atmospheric air, of preventing the slow oxidation of phosphorus, which renders it luminous in the dark. He found that olefiant gas, and the vapour of oil of turpentine, and of other essential oils, possess this power, even when present in a very minute quantity. I expressed an opinion nearly five years ago,‡ that the action of ether on the human frame was of the same kind as that by which it prevented the oxidation of phosphorus; and this view is supported by the fact, that amongst substances of a similar constitution, whose narcotic power is known, this power bears a direct relation to the power of preventing the oxidation of phosphorus. For example, I find that the vapour of alcohol has but little influence in this respect, whilst Prof. Graham found that the vapour of ether, in the proportion of one part to 150 of air, prevents the oxidation of phosphorus at all temperatures up to 64° Faht.; that one part of olefiant gas (which is a more powerful narcotic) has a like effect in 450 parts of air; and that one part of vapour of naphtha exerts this influence when diluted with 1820 parts of air. Now naphtha consists chiefly of benzin, which, as was stated in a former paper, causes insensibility when less than a grain of it it diffused in each hundred cubic inches of the

---

* I am persuaded that the antiseptic properties of various substances are capable of producing greater advantages than they have hitherto, especially if applied by the method of injecting the arteries immediately after death, which was described in my last paper. Owing to the difficulty of curing meat by the ordinary methods in tropical climates, thousands of oxen and sheep are slaughtered in South America and Australia, for the tallow and hides, whilst the flesh is left to rot; when, by injecting the vessels, it could be immediately rendered as firm as in the coldest climate. There would probably be a prejudice against using a medicine such as chloroform for this purpose; but it fortunately happens that the essential oils, which exist in nearly all condiments, are both narcotic and antiseptic. I have frequently made insects insensible by exposing them in a covered vessel to the vapour of oil of peppermint; and, on one occasion, I rendered a linnet insensible by the inhalation of the vapour of oil of lemons: by injecting twenty minims only of the latter essential oil (shaken up with an ounce of water) into the arteries of a rabbit after death, it kept very well for seventeen days. I have found that injecting with a saturated solution of common salt very much hastens rigidity, although it does not produce it immediately. I hope that some one who has the opportunity will follow up this subject, as it promises to yield a kind of wealth more useful than the newly-discovered treasures of California and Australia.

* Quarterly Jour. of Sc., 1829, part ii. p. 354.
† Op. cit.
‡ See MED. GAZ., vol. xxxix. p. 383.

respired air. Professor Graham ascertained that hydrochloric acid gas promotes the oxidation of phosphorus in the air; and I find that the vapour of chloroform does not prevent it: this is probably due to the chlorine it contains in such large quantity.

Professor Graham states that olefiant gas prevents phosphorus and hydrogen from uniting with oxygen without undergoing any change itself. This is exactly analogous to the action of ether and chloroform in the human body, which, as shown before, produce their effects, and pass off unchanged in the expired air.

Having traced the narcotic action of ether and other bodies to the more general law of their power of preventing oxidation under a great variety of circumstances, the mind naturally inquires by what kind of power oxidation is thus prevented. I feel considerable diffidence in offering a theory on a subject which falls as much within the domain of ordinary chemistry, as within that of physiology, when so eminent a chemist as Professor Graham has investigated a number of its details without suggesting any general explanation on the matter. However, as I have formed a theory in my own mind, I offer it for consideration: it is to the following effect :—That chemical attraction or affinity is a constantly acting force, by which each atom of matter exerts an influence on all other atoms within the sphere of its attraction, whether they are of the same or of a different kind, the force of the attraction varying with the respective nature of the substances, and the physical conditions in which they are placed. In this point of view, it will be seen that any two substances in a condition to unite together might be prevented from doing so by the intervention of a third body possessing a sufficient attraction for either of the others; and it would not be necessary that this third body should itself enter into chemical combination; for a balance of forces might be established, so that the three substances would remain exerting reciprocal attractions for each other, but unable to enter into more intimate union.

In the instances of prevented oxidation previously considered, the interfering substances no doubt owe their influence to their attraction for oxygen.

These substances, in fact, are known to possess a strong affinity for oxygen, being nearly all of them highly combustible. Those of them which have the greatest power in preventing oxidation—as olefiant gas and benzin—contain no oxygen in their composition; whilst the oxide of ethyle, which contains rather more than one fifth of its weight of oxygen, has less power; and alcohol, which consists of oxygen to the extent of rather more than one-third, has much less power than ether as a narcotic, as an antiseptic, and in preventing the oxidation of phosphorus. The salts of ethyle, without oxygen, produce narcotic effects also in much smaller doses than its oxygen salts. It was previously shown that the narcotic powers of the ethers and other allied agents was in the inverse ratio of their solubility in water,—a generalization which is in perfect accordance with what is now stated; for it so happens that the agents of this class which contain oxygen are more soluble than those which do not.

As regards their application to the substances when acting as narcotics, the views just explained may be thus briefly stated. When absorbed into the blood, they have an attraction for the oxygen dissolved in it; and though unable to combine with the oxygen under the circumstances, the attraction is sufficient to counteract that existing between the oxygen, on the one hand, and certain constituents of the blood and tissues of the organs, on the other; and thus the combinations between the respired oxygen and the materials of the body—those changes which are, in a manner, the essence of all the animal functions—are prevented more or less completely, according to the dose of the narcotic.

There is a curious circumstance connected with the oxidation of phosphorus, to which it is necessary to allude. Professor Graham found that pure oxygen has no action on phosphorus under the atmospheric pressure, at temperatures below 64°; but that a slight expansion of the gas, by diminishing the pressure two or three inches, or diluting the oxygen with nitrogen, hydrogen, or certain other gases, enables it to act on the phosphorus, which then becomes luminous in the dark. The explanation I would offer of this circumstance is, that the attraction or affinity of the atoms of oxygen for each other is sufficient to prevent their combining with the phosphorus until that attraction is weakened by their separation to a greater distance by the diminution of the pressure or the intervention of the atoms of another gas.

In dismissing this part of the subject I should like to remark, that whatever may be thought of the above explanation of the power by which certain narcotics retard or arrest oxidation in the animal frame, will not affect the fact of these narcotics acting in this way, for it rests on distinct evidence previously stated.

I have said nothing of the stimulant or irritant properties which chloroform, ether, alcohol, and probably all narcotics, possess in a greater or less degree, and I have not space to enter on that subject; but I expect to be able to show on another occasion, that the irritation caused by narcotics is not opposed to the view of their acting in the way explained in the previous pages.

These papers on narcotism by the inhalation of vapours have extended over a very much longer time than I expected, and I have done after all much less than I intended. In now bringing them to a close, however, it may be well to give a brief recapitulation of the more prominent points which I have endeavoured to establish.

Several experiments with chloroform and ether were described, the object of which was to determine the quantity of these agents which exists in the blood in a state of insensibility. The method employed was that of placing a small animal in a large vessel, containing a known quantity of vapour mixed with the air, and allowing it to remain till the effects of the vapour no longer increased, but became stationary; when, the solubility of the vapour in the serum of the blood being known, the quantity absorbed could be calculated from the relative saturation of the air. It was found that, with both chloroform and ether, the proportion, in a state of complete insensibility, was about one twenty-eighth part as much as the blood would dissolve. Similar experiments were made with several other substances, including some salts of ethyle, benzin, bromoform, Dutch liquid, and sulphuret of carbon, and it was found that the proportion absorbed into the blood, in causing insensibility, was nearly the same as in the case of ether or chloroform. Hence the rule was deduced, that the narcotic strength of these substances was in the inverse ratio of their solubility. The agents to which this rule applies resemble chloroform and ether in containing carbon, and not containing any nitrogen as a radical element, and some of them were used as was described with success, in preventing the pain of surgical operations.

A description of the influence of chloroform was given, in which the effects it produces, if continued until respiration is suspended, were divided into five degrees. It was stated that when chloroform is given to animals neither very quickly nor slowly, and continued till the breathing is arrested, the heart continues to beat; but some experiments were detailed which show that chloroform is capable of arresting the action of the heart, if absorbed in sufficient quantity.

The cases of accident from inhalation of chloroform, which had happened up to the time of writing, were next considered, when it appeared that the fatal event in these cases was due to the vapour of chloroform being given in too concentrated a form, by which not only was the breathing suddenly arrested, but the action of the heart was also paralysed by the effect of the vapour.*

The opinion was expressed that chloroform, if given gradually and with due care, may be safely employed in every case in which a surgical operation has to be performed; an opinion in which I have been altogether confirmed by further experience.

Directions were next given for the administration of chloroform in various kinds of operations; the conditions and diatheses which influence its action were considered, and a numerical result of the larger operations in which I had administered chloroform or ether at that

* The fatal cases which have since happened, together with some that narrowly escaped being fatal, entirely confirm the opinion then expressed. The alarming symptoms always came on in the most sudden manner, the action of the heart being suspended without previous warning, although in some of the cases there had been at first an apparent difficulty in rendering the patient insensible. No means were used in any of these cases to insure a proper dilution of the vapour with air, a handkerchief being merely employed for administering chloroform, except I believe in one case, where it was not administered by a medical man.

time was given, by which it was shown that the result had been favourable.

After some remarks on the use of Dutch liquid in operations and mid wifery, some experiments with alcohol were detailed, by which it was shown to resemble ether and chloroform in its effects and mode of action. Experiments were related showing that chloro form passes off unchanged in the expired air; that it can be detected in limbs amputated whilst patients are inhaling, and also in the dead bodies of animals killed by it. It was next shown that ether and alcohol can be detected in the expired air, and that the quantity of carbonic acid excreted by the lungs is diminished under the influence of chloroform and ether. For these and other reasons the conclusion was arrived at, that the class of narcotics we have been considering, and probably other narcotics also, produce their effects by virtue of a power they possess of retarding the action of the respired oxygen on the blood and tissues of the body.

54, Frith Street, Soho Square.

Index

Index

nitric ether   13
 anaesthesia, Snow anticipates further
   study of   14
 blood levels of and degrees of
   narcotism   15
 Dr Simpson's views on   14
 in dogs   14
 Snow determines approx. Specific
   Gravity of   13
 Snow gives to a patient   14
 Snow inhales it himself   14
 Snow predicts the safety of in anaes-
   thesia   14
nitrogen, carburet of   96
Norway   14
Nottingham   54
Nottingham General Hospital, the   54
Nunnelly, Mr   59
 praises Dutch Liquid   65
Nysten   94

Ogston, Dr   69
olefiant gas   18, 97
 anti-explosive effect of   97
 anti-oxidant effect of   98
On Bromine and its Compounds
 (Glover)   17
*On the Inhalation of the Vapour of
 Ether* (Snow)   23
On the Presence of Alcohol in the brain
 (Dr Percy)   78
onlookers/friends present during
 operations   42
opium
 Battley's solution of   56
 treatment of vomiting with   56
Osnaburg Street   63
oxidation, effects of anaesthetic agents
 on   91
oxygen
 for cholera, Snow's use of   80
 injection into heart's cavities, effects
   of   94
oxygen lack, as a mechanism for
 anaesthesia, Snow repudiates   70
oxygenation, venous, effects of anaesthesia on   94
pain
 chloroform and post-operative   45
 Snow's definition of   22
pamphlet on chloroform in the practice
 of midwifery (Dr Murphy)   20
Paris   13, 96
 alleged chloroform fatality in   30

Hôpital Beaujon   30
 the Hospitals of   47
Parkinson, Mr   62
Parrott, Mr John   76
Pearson, Mrs, account of a chloroform
 fatality by   28
Percy Dr   78–9
 *On the Presence of Alcohol in the
   Brain*   78
Pereira, Dr   60
phagadena, post-operative, sloughing
 42
phosphorus, ability of anaesthetics to
 prevent oxidation of   97
Physicians, the College of   9
Physiological Researches (Sir B Brodie)
 94
Pollock, Mr George   53
polyps, operations for nasal   52
Portugal Street No. 10, Lincoln's Inn
 Fields   33
position
 patient's, during operation and
   anaesthesia   35
 for amputations   44
potency of vapours varies inversely
 with their solubility in blood   19
pre-filled balloon
 use of, as an inhaler   59
 use of, for mixture of different
   volatile agents   59
pregnancy, effects of chloroform
 in   43
preservation of meat, Snow's views on
 use of narcotics for the   97
Price, Mr   14
Prout, Dr   85, 93
pulse
 changes in during anaesthesia   23
 no indication of the degree of narcotism   23
putrefaction
 effects of anaesthetics on   96
 M Robin's views on   96
 retarded by antiseptics and narcotics
   87
pyroxilic spirit (wood naphtha)   19
 experiments on fishes with   68

Read, the late Mr (instrument maker)
 68
Regnault, M   60
Regnault, Mons V   81
Reiset, Mons J   81

[**110**]